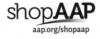
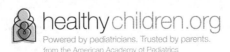

The Baby Bonding Book

Connecting With Your Newborn

Joanna Parga-Belinkie, MD, FAAP, IBCLC

American Academy of Pediatrics

DEDICATED TO THE HEALTH OF ALL CHILDREN®

American Academy of Pediatrics Publishing Staff

Mark Grimes, *Vice President, Publishing*

Jeff Mahony, *Senior Director, Professional and Consumer Publishing*

Holly Kaminski, *Editor, Consumer Publishing*

Jason Crase, *Senior Manager, Production and Editorial Services*

Shannan Martin, *Production Manager, Consumer Publications*

Soraya Alem, *Manager, Digital Publishing*

Sara Hoerdeman, *Marketing and Acquisitions Manager, Consumer Products*

Published by the American Academy of Pediatrics
345 Park Blvd
Itasca, IL 60143
Telephone: 630/626-6000
Facsimile: 847/434-8000
www.aap.org

The American Academy of Pediatrics is an organization of 67,000 primary care pediatricians, pediatric medical subspecialists, and pediatric surgical specialists dedicated to the health, safety, and well-being of all infants, children, adolescents, and young adults.

The information contained in this publication should not be used as a substitute for the medical care and advice of your pediatrician. There may be variations in treatment that your pediatrician may recommend based on individual facts and circumstances.

Statements and opinions expressed are those of the author and not necessarily those of the American Academy of Pediatrics.

Any websites, brand names, products, or manufacturers are mentioned for informational and identification purposes only and do not imply an endorsement by the American Academy of Pediatrics (AAP). The AAP is not responsible for the content of external resources. Information was current at the time of publication.

The publishers have made every effort to trace the copyright holders for borrowed materials. If they have inadvertently overlooked any, they will be pleased to make the necessary arrangements at the first opportunity.

This publication has been developed by the American Academy of Pediatrics. The contributors are expert authorities in the field of pediatrics. No commercial involvement of any kind has been solicited or accepted in the development of the content of this publication. Disclosures: The author reports no disclosures.

Every effort is made to keep *The Baby Bonding Book: Connecting With Your Newborn* consistent with the most recent advice and information available from the American Academy of Pediatrics.

Special discounts are available for bulk purchases of this publication. Email Special Sales at nationalaccounts@aap.org for more information.

Printed in the United States of America

9-516   1 2 3 4 5 6 7 8 9 10

CB0141

ISBN: 978-1-61002-785-4

eBook: 978-1-61002-786-1

EPUB: 978-1-61002-787-8

Cover and publication design by Scott Rattray Design

Library of Congress Control Number: 2024941849

WHAT PEOPLE ARE SAYING ABOUT
THE BABY BONDING BOOK

All it takes is to read a few sentences, and you will find yourself strongly bonding with *The Baby Bonding Book*. Using evidence-based scientific knowledge combined with lived experience, humor, humility, and an unconditional love for building the most meaningful parent-infant relationship possible, Dr Parga-Belinkie has written a volume that makes you feel like you are getting expert advice written specifically for you and your baby!

> Lewis First, MD, MS, FAAP, professor and chair, Department of Pediatrics, University of Vermont Robert Larner, MD College of Medicine; chief of pediatrics, University of Vermont Children's Hospital; and editor in chief, *Pediatrics*

As a pediatrician, I am a baby expert. But when I have a question about babies, especially newborns or babies born prematurely, I call Dr Joanna Parga-Belinkie. In addition to being a pediatrician, she is a neonatologist, meaning that caring for babies is all she does day and night in her job at arguably the number 1 children's hospital in the world. That's not all, though. She's also a mom 3 times over, and she addresses the problems that parents face with an empathy that can only come from working through so many of them herself. Now you, too, can enjoy Joanna's expertise, her warmth, her humor, and her understanding of the struggles involved in birth and parenting a new baby. What's happening to your body? Your emotions? Your baby's everything, from tummy to brain? Dr Parga-Belinkie provides answers and, even better, comfort.

> David L. Hill, MD, FAAP, author of *Dad to Dad: Parenting Like a Pro*, associate medical editor of *Caring for Your Baby and Young Child: Birth to Age 5*, and adjunct associate professor of pediatrics at the UNC School of Medicine

As a neonatologist and pediatrician, I highly recommend *The Baby Bonding Book* by Dr Parga-Belinkie. With a warm, relatable voice, she reassures new parents that they already have the instincts and love needed to nurture their baby—while providing evidence-based guidance to build a secure, loving bond amid the challenges of early parenthood.

> Ashley D. Osborne, MD, FAAP, assistant professor of pediatrics and neonatologist, Medical University of South Carolina

PLEASE NOTE

The author respects and acknowledges the diversity and range of the gender spectrum and gender identity. Please note that for the entirety of this book, when we refer to "girls" and "women" we are referencing those who identify as female. When we refer to "boys" and "men" we are referencing those who identify as male. We recognize those individuals who self-identify as a gender other than their sex assignment at birth, and those for whom their gender is fluid.

This book is dedicated to the 3 "babies" I share my home with. I hope our relationship can be a model for how you shape the many relationships you will love and cherish in your lifetime. And to my littlest Baby Z who I was pregnant with when I wrote this, carrying you through the experience of writing a book about babies was very meta. Your conception and birth were the bookends to this creation, and the joy you bring this family could fill pages.

EQUITY, DIVERSITY, AND INCLUSION STATEMENT

The American Academy of Pediatrics is committed to principles of equity, diversity, and inclusion in its publishing program. Editorial boards, author selections, and author transitions (publication succession plans) are designed to include diverse voices that reflect society as a whole. Editor and author teams are encouraged to actively seek out diverse authors and reviewers at all stages of the editorial process. Publishing staff are committed to promoting equity, diversity, and inclusion in all aspects of publication writing, review, and production.

Contents

Foreword

Why do we love? So people know they are worthy of being loved.[1]

Why do we protect? So people know they deserve to feel safe.

Why do we listen? So people know they should be heard.

My work is focused on supporting adults to be the kind of people their children deserve in their lives. It's an easy job because people want to be that kind of adult. We all want healthy family relationships that will endure through adolescence and beyond.

One more "why." Why am I, a pediatrician who primarily serves adolescents and their families, writing the foreword to a book about bonding with your newborn? Because your relationship begins on day 1. It is forever forged the second your newborn grasps your finger and senses you are someone uniquely special in their lives. The moment you realize your heart is now on the outside of your body, you are forever committed to being a protective force in their life.

Dr Joanna Parga-Belinkie guides you to notice the signals your infant is sending as a first step to knowing them. She says, for example, "One great way to nurture is by listening when your baby has something to say." Exactly!! Babies don't talk, but they communicate.

---

1   I first heard this question, and its strikingly clear answer, from Kevin Ryan, formerly the CEO of Covenant House International.

They speak in a language that only their parents learn to understand because of an unwavering commitment to respond to—and meet—their baby's needs. This sets the tone for our relationship. We'll show up. *We'll let our children know from the very first days that we know they should be listened to.* As Dr. Joanna says, "An infant wants to express themselves and be heard; they want to have someone respond to them."

I love this book because while it offers practical how-to guidance, its essence is about building a nurturant relationship between you and the little human who has come into your life. I love this book because it doesn't pretend building that relationship is easy or straightforward. Just very, very important. I love this book because it gives you permission to feel confused about how to build that relationship and to experience frustration along the journey.

This book is so accessible because it offers tips with a healthy dose of—sometimes disarming—humor. I know Joanna and I'll tell you that she's really that funny in person. More importantly, she's deeply serious. Humor—even a bit of sarcasm—makes it easy to learn the vitally important stuff. It is ok to laugh at ourselves sometimes. Dr Joanna sets the tone by laughing at herself and some of the missteps she has taken in her own journey.

We must be intentional to try to get it right but to not be too hard on ourselves when we don't. In fact, let me reassure you that the finest humans are raised by . . . humans. Fallible, complex, often bewildered humans. Humans who fumble and are willing to grow from their mistakes. Humans who are willing to turn to others for support and guidance when they don't yet possess the answers. Seekers. Humans who understand that the details aren't what matters—it is our connection that offers those we care about a sense of belonging. And that is what makes the difference. Because let's be honest, perfect people are terrible role models.

Strive to be a good role model.

This book speaks of nurturance as the root of safety. Babies really are helpless, so we all know we must keep them physically safe. Here, you will be able to reflect on the root of psychological safety. Dr Joanna says that such safety is ". . . the ability to interact with others and say what you really feel and mean without fear that something bad will happen to you." This book guides you to let your infant express themselves and learn from them how you can best address their needs. Now is not the time to have them tough it out. This is the time you instill within them the deep-seated knowledge of how profoundly and unconditionally they are loved. That they matter. That is the root of resilience.

Fast-forward: We know the kind of parental style that forges the type of relationships that will position you to best guide your child through the school years, adolescence, and beyond. It is about striking that balance of nurturance (expressed love) and demandingness (discipline and rules). The scientific literature calls this *authoritative parenting*. Your great grandparents called it common sense. I call it Lighthouse Parenting. You are a stable, present guide. You protect from danger. But you prepare them to navigate the world on their own. You'll always be there; when they trust they can ride the waves on their own, they'll choose to return to you.

We know that this style of parenting builds the best relationships, the kind where children seek parental involvement in their lives. It creates the most emotionally secure children and adolescents with the lowest behavioral risks. It also produces children and teens with the best academic performance to boot! Again . . . and again . . . the roots of relationship start on day 1. You can never be too nurturant. Too much love has never spoiled a child. It makes them sweeter. Critically, your unconditional and unwavering love makes them more receptive to your protective guidance. You *can* be too demanding. The secret is to serve as a guide and to understand that preparation is the very best protection. Bubble Wrap; not an option. And yes, you must draw the line clearly and absolutely around safety issues—not because you want to control them, but because you love them. *Remember, you want to instill in your child the knowledge that they deserve to feel physically and emotionally safe.*

Whoa, Dr Ken, my child isn't taking solid foods yet, I have to think about all of this . . . now?!?!? Yes, let Dr Joanna guide you *now* about nurturant connections. That bond will last forever. But don't be demanding now. As a tiny little thing, it's your infant's turn to practice being demanding with you! When you let them be the boss of you—for now—they'll gain the deep-seated sense of security that comes from understanding when they ask for their needs to get met, someone is listening. Trust me, later when you need to be setting the rules, they'll be more likely to be followed because they'll trust it comes from a place of genuine caring.

Congratulations on your newborn. There are a lot of details to parenting. None of us get them all right. But do what really counts the most. *Raise a human who knows without question they are worthy of being loved.*

KENNETH GINSBURG, MD, MSEd, FAAP

Author of

Building Resilience in Children and Teens: Giving Kids Roots and Wings

Lighthouse Parenting: Raising Your Child With Loving Guidance for a Lifelong Bond

And you're not ready for this one . . . yet 😊

Congrats—You're Having a Teen! Strengthen Your Family and Raise a Good Person

Acknowledgments

Wissahickon Valley State Park is a beautiful nature preserve unexpectedly blossoming on the edge of the city of Philadelphia. I was walking through the canopy of greenery and over rushing waterways on winding trails when Dr Kenneth Ginsberg encouraged me to write a book. He suggested it while we were watching a family of ducks diving in and out of a pond at the end of our hike. This was for me a career-altering meeting surrounded by nature, and I'll never forget how transformative it was. Thank you for pushing me to put myself on paper and for making me spell out my love for babies and bonding with them. And a special thank you to the family of ducks that helped me find whimsy and strength when thinking about the serious topics of relationships and love. Thanks to American Academy of Pediatrics (AAP) Publishing for taking a chance on my stories and my humor—without you seeing me I would not have become an author. And thank you to the many groups at the AAP that gave suggestions and their knowledge and wisdom to this text.

Stable, safe, and nurturing relationships made this book possible. Mom and Dad—you were always nurturing me. While being a family means there are times things aren't always stable or safe, you have always loved and supported me, and I carry that love with me every single day. To my husband Danny—you are so many things to our family. A self-proclaimed realist, and a calming laid-back and go with the flow force. We have similar values but different parenting styles. Learning about love with you for a lifetime is a treat and an honor. I wouldn't want to do this with anyone else. And to the many friends that listened to the title, helped shape chapters, and encouraged me—I want you to know how much you helped me. Without your guidance and support none of this would be possible.

Introduction

"People love giving pregnant women advice, don't they? They love it. The whole time I was pregnant, I have this one friend, she'd always tell me, she's like, 'You have to do prenatal yoga. It really helps with the birth. Prenatal yoga.' So I immediately signed up for a c-section."

AMY SCHUMER, EMERGENCY CONTACT

*B*eing pregnant means, all of a sudden, people have a lot of advice and thoughts for you. I was pregnant with my third baby and working full time. I had just started feeling better after 2 straight months of moderate nausea and vomiting, which included excusing myself from deliveries to go to the bathroom and throw up. Once I was so nauseous I had to throw up in a hospital hallway sink. I was almost banished from my shift for concerns I had a stomach bug. I was disappointed, but I had to let everyone around me know that I was 9 weeks' pregnant. Most times though I worked through all the stomach upset desperately trying to hide the fact I was harboring a fetus. Somehow though when you spend a lot of time in the bathroom, look pale, and occasionally attempt to nap on the overmopped hospital floor...people notice. I remember someone telling me after I revealed my pregnancy in the second trimester, "I knew something was up, you looked really bad, like something was wrong with you."

I had been sick with my other pregnancies too, but it was much worse with my last one. Being pregnant when your job is a neonatol-

ogist—or baby doctor—I imagine opens you up to more comments on your appearance than the average pregnant woman. I am typically surrounded by pregnant or immediately postpartum women every day at work. My whole job is dealing with birth and babies. I remember I was climbing the stairs after having to run to a delivery in the third trimester of my pregnancy. On the way back to the neonatal intensive care unit (NICU), I took my time step by step, already feeling like I was carrying a lot. I was out of breath when I reached the NICU. One of the hospital employees saw me walk by and stopped me.

"Are you ok?" she said.

"Yeah, just a little out of breath."

"Yeah you are really showing. Are you sure there is just one baby in there?"

Yes, I was very sure. The comment made me feel uneasy. It wasn't the first or last time I was asked if I were carrying multiple babies. In those moments I would feel pressure to explain myself and my pregnancy— things that were private health matters. I'm usually very open, but I went through a lot to have my last baby including fertility treatments and many months of heartache.

Discussion about a pregnant person's body is often unproductive and can leave them feeling vulnerable and defensive. Asking me if I was having twins brought up so much about my pregnancy journey and the struggles to have just one baby. Those comments on my size made me feel bad about myself, like I looked massive and was out of shape (… you try exercising in between having to vomit every other day…). In reality I was trying really hard to be healthy—I walked a ton, ate a balanced diet, and expended a lot of energy chasing my other 2 kids. For each of my pregnancies, I gained the same amount of weight. It helped me realize how many things were out of my control. I was not focusing on an ideal pregnancy body, but my goal was to have healthy habits for me and my fetus while I was pregnant.

Reflecting on becoming pregnant after you have been trying, or planning, or dreaming about this day can be such an amazing moment to experience. Pregnancy itself is a journey filled with checkups, ultrasounds, and bloodwork, and it is a public reminder to those around you that there is a baby inside you. It's no wonder when you are pregnant you feel like you have to have answers and explainations for what's going on with your body. You will get unwanted attention or comments about your changing physique and you will think you have to answer for that. Luckily, though, most people are kind. They will see you as a whole. People will understand you are going through something and most want to be there for you. However, because of the chatter and commentary surrounding pregnancy, I've found more and more families are creating a birth plan for their delivery. They want to imagine what the moment will be like when the baby arrives. They have a playlist ready to go, have researched the medications they want, and have a ton of expectations and nerves about how their changing body will perform in the moment.

Those feelings of excitement and anticipation grow, and your baby finally arrives. Then, very quickly your mood may switch to feeling overwhelmed. All that time spent on those thoughts and feelings of the excitement for your baby's arrival are slowly fading now that they are here and you are going to have to take them home. In the midst of changing hormones and a new life, the postpartum period has taken you off guard. How do you take care of this little one? How will you bond with them? Why do you feel exhausted and maybe a little sad? What do you do when they cry? And how do you know what information to trust for their care?

Because the hope is pregnancy ends with a new person who will be a major part of your family. Planning for the birth is important because it is a huge moment and you can feel like you are pregnant FOREVER. The truth is, though, forever really happens afterward when you have delivered this new person into the world and have to parent them for the rest of your life.

But what do you really know about your baby? How do you get to know your baby? What strategies are you going to use to establish a *close connection with your newborn? What are your goals for parenting a newborn? Were you supposed to have goals for that?!?!*

> *"You're just in solitary confinement all day long with this human Tamagotchi…[who doesn't have any] reset button, so the stakes are extremely high. A toy Tamagotchi is more communicative than a human baby. Okay? Because the toy will at least tell you when it poos."*
>
> ALI WONG, *Hard Knock Wife*

In preparation for the baby, most families have made lists of boy and girl names and have selected a baby name or two. Maybe the nursery is decorated. They might have a cute outfit to take the baby home in, a photoshoot planned for right after they leave the hospital. Maybe they have started to create that baby announcement to send to friends and family but are waiting to find out if it will be pink or blue lettering. However, what I see few families consider is the *who* of their baby. This new person you have created, who will be entering the world, what will they be like? What will their personality be, or their temperament? On top of that, how will this new baby change *you*? It might be time to consider how you are going to bond with this new person to figure out a way to get to know your infant and build a relationship with this tiny person you created.

Because, let's be honest, no one else is going to be thinking about your relationship with the baby and how you will change except for those close to you. Other people stop seeing you as pregnant and don't realize how much your world begins to change. Like delivering the baby was the big deal, and now it's back to business as usual. They will ask about how the baby is doing but not necessarily how *you* are doing or how you are feeling. There will be some bizarre expectation that within a few months you'll have lost all the baby weight. Without the baby inside you, somehow it will be easy to

return to "the before times." It's like without the physical reminder
of the new baby, society forgets that it's even harder on you once the
baby is delivered because that baby now needs needs your unwavering love, support, time, and attention. Despite, perhaps, not knowing
how to connect, or being intimidated by them, you connect with
your baby, discover the person you want to raise, and let yourself
grow in the process. That is why baby bonding time is essential—why
you have to shift the focus a little from how you will physically feel
and recover, to thinking about the relationship you want to have with
your new child.

Not knowing your baby before delivery means you aren't going
to know what kind of parent you will be. Maybe you've already
settled into the mindset you will be super strict or extra permissive,
or you've already rented a helicopter because there is no way baby is
going to crawl without a cadre of parental aerial support. Before you
make assumptions about what it's going to be like with your baby,
consider that this person is a complete stranger. Right after birth, you
finally come face to face with a new human being. Before delivery,
you don't even really know what their birth weight will be! A friend
of mine brought a spectacular onesie to the hospital, excitedly thinking it was a going home outfit. But when her baby shocked everyone
and weighed 9 pounds, the newborn size didn't fit them and the
outfit was never worn. The onesie was replaced by a white hospital
shirt wrap with diaper showing, and there are professional photos
commemorating the fact that this baby had nothing cute to wear.
The big baby was not what my friend was expecting but was what she
got. Your personal stranger (ie, new baby) is destined to surprise you.
They will immediately move into your house, share a room with you,
and place their survival in your hands. If they could speak (or even
just understand words), you'd be able to set some boundaries early
on and express how awkward it is that you will be bunking together
for the next 18+ years without even so much as a personality test or

an interview. But you don't get that sort of face time with an infant; it's more skin to skin, which is a very important way to communicate with your baby. The language of newborns is based on hormones, crying, and context cues. To form a relationship with your infant, you're going to have to adapt to a new way of listening, speaking, and learning (and, of course, poop smelling).

I know this because I spend much of my day job trying to decode what infants are thinking, how they are feeling, and ways to uncover their budding personality. My medical training is all about babies. I spend most of the time in a NICU. My formal education has centered around preterm or sick babies. I'll admit it is different to take care of a healthy baby. There are no vital sign machines, no x-rays, no laboratory studies to follow. But somehow, parents learn to care for their babies. You will too. Caring for babies has been a practice long before the profession of neonatology was founded: before smartphones, diaper-counting apps, or self-rocking cribs. Because to truly care for a newborn, you have to get to know them. Infants have a hardwired temperament that follows them throughout their lives, and you are just along for the ride. So let's get to know your baby.

Relationship Building With a Newborn

How are you going to build a lifelong relationship with arguably the most important person you will ever know? Relationships are tricky. My relationship with my husband was one of the most profound ones I worked on before having children. When I told my parents I was going to marry an artist, they questioned my love for him. Couldn't I just fall for another doctor? (It is reported that 1 in 4 female physicians marry other doctors.) What's a grip? (My husband used to be a grip, or, as he put it, the "gorilla" of a film set. The person behind the scenes setting up lights. Not very gripping as it turns out. Now he's a cinematographer and focuses on filming.) Are you sure that's a job? (Yes, I'm sure a grip is a job, so is a "best boy," second assistant director, and Foley artist). Although some may question your love for your partner, no one will question the love you have for your baby. You can choose to express that love in any number of ways. For some, it may be the first time you are "allowed" to love someone you just met. That instinctual, unconditional love will push you to the edges of your sanity—and beyond. Does this sound crazy? It is.

While people won't question your love for the baby, they will have a lot of questions and comments about your parenting style. It's no wonder new parents feel like they already have to *know every-thing*. Oh, you aren't breastfeeding? You *know* it's one the best things you could possibly do for your infant, right? Haven't you heard of water wipes? I see the ones you are using contain preservatives; don't you *know* those are bad? Why didn't you think of getting a pee-pee teepee? I don't *know* if you *know*, but the exchange of bodily fluids is about to get real and don't you want to be prepared?

How should you as a parent react to this barrage of well-intentioned advice seemingly aimed at making you anxious? Let me tell you about something certified baby doctors (aka neonatologists) often question. When a baby exits the womb, we cannot decide if they are 0 or 1 day old. Ultimately, I've settled on the logic that you can't be 0 days old. Being 8 hours old means you are 1 day old. But sure, if you are 8 hours old, you are 0 full days old. So, I see where the zero-ists have a case. If experts can't agree on how old an infant is on arrival, how can they agree about more important topics surrounding newborns? Things like feeding, sleep, pacifiers, and reflux. No one likes to experiment on newborns, so finding definitive answers for newborn issues is a true challenge. This leads to a lot of *opinions* about newborn care. That said, life is a great natural experiment. We might not agree on the age of a newborn, but neonatal and pediatric experts do agree about *important things*. Topics we can and do study to give infants a healthy start for the long and enduring relationship you are about to build with them. I'll share those with you, all the other things I wanted to give my baby after delivery to help them thrive.

When the well-meaning advice starts to come, just say you are still figuring out what works for *your* baby and *your* relationship with them. You knew breastfeeding was an option, but maybe for you it truly wasn't the best choice because anatomically, emotionally, or medically it wasn't possible for you. So far, your baby has not had a reaction to the generic baby wipes you purchased, so you're going to finish them up and then decide if you want to switch. You've never heard of a pee-pee teepee? Admit it, don't fret over it (it's a tent that goes over a penis to stop urine from spraying everywhere when you change the baby's diaper). The reason you haven't heard of it yet is because it's optional. While optional can be meaningful, you don't *need* it for the health and safety of your infant. A dry washcloth or an extra wipe of your choosing does the same job of stopping a urine fountain from spraying everywhere.

It's important to center yourself on what really matters: an infant's connection to you, their loving attentive caregiver. The attachment you have to your infant will help shape them biochemically into the person they will become. The newborn period is fleeting, and in that brief time you will begin to understand the essential role you play as a parent in just being present. Does that mean just loving them and hanging out with them is all they need to grow and thrive? No, if only it were that simple. You are going to be called upon to make decisions affecting their health and safety. I want to help you cut through the noise of infant care and get to the literal heart of it. I want you to love being with your newborn and cherish every uncertainty that comes with building a relationship and parenting a nonverbal human in a safe and supported way. Let's embrace our babies and get to bonding with them!

Chapter 1

Running to the Start Line: Parenting Before Baby Arrives

My baby registry for my first baby included a lot things. Somehow, I felt if I had the equipment lined up to care for my child, I'd be ready. I gathered others' baby registries, cross-referencing theirs with the list I was creating. Because I had a plan and all this stuff, it was going to save me from the common pitfalls of baby rearing. It was going to make parenting **easier** for me. This led to the accumulation of what I felt I needed to be prepared. It was the little mermaid approach to parenting. Thingamabobs? I've got 20! But who cares, no big deal, I wanted more. I somehow felt my collection of products related to my parenting was the first step to parenting.

As it turns out, when you are a trained pediatrician and neonatologist who has a bunch of purchased items from your baby registry organized around your house, you have not won the parenting game. I in fact have yet to win the mom of the year award (who gives that out anyway?) because it was not based on my bomb baby registry and a premier baby lounger as recommended by my targeted internet ads. It was helpful to have a diaper station set up and a safe sleep space, but aside from a few key items (diapers, ample onesies, and a safe sleep surface), nothing I bought was going to make me parent better. My first daughter cried uncontrollably every evening when she was a few weeks old. During those harrowing 90-minute scream fests—commonly dubbed the witching hour (picture the sea witch Ursula laughing maniacally as my baby let out a bunch of ah-ah-ahhs and my husband and I the poor unfortunate souls)—I abandoned every item I purchased from *my baby registry and was forced to rely on myself and the other humans around me. No mermaids were available to participate. Ultimately, my husband or I would just carry her around until the screaming subsided. Why did I want to be a part of this world again? I was not wandering free, and there were other places I definitely wished I could be.*

Here is one challenge with parenting a newborn: Before they are even born, you can be overwhelmed by numerous targeted baby products, good intentions, and ample advice. But parenting really means just being a loving, attentive, grown-up presence for your child—there is little fanfare in doing that. You need to have confidence that you are enough. That might come with having babies, but I'll just tell you this: YOU ARE EVERYTHING TO YOUR BABY. Take some time to think about the big picture: Who is this person I want to raise? What should I do to prepare myself for this responsibility? How might this new task change me? Instead of fretting about the day-to-day monotony that accompanies caring for newborns, focus on your bigger vision and goals for the person you want to share your life with; the other stuff then won't seem as cumbersome. Because you are envisioning the relationship you want to have with the person you are growing to love.

Before Baby Bonding: Understanding Parenting

To prepare yourself to parent a newborn is to understand you are everything this baby needs. For your baby, you are going to be the sun, moon, stars, sky, grass, trees, and the darn dirt. This can be an overwhelming or even an unbelievable realization for a new parent. When the baby finally arrives, many parents think they have to be doing something with them every minute of the day to help them thrive. What you need to realize is that just being there next to them—holding them, talking to them, and rocking them—is what really counts and is the only activity your newborn needs.

Before the baby's debut, take a big breath, in through your nose and out through your mouth. Ok, do it again. Now picture yourself just holding your new infant. Yes, their survival and development are going to be driven by you, but all your baby wants is you. Start to imagine yourself as being comfortable in the brief moments of stillness when holding a newborn. The quiet times, no cell phone, no TV, no guests: just you and your newborn. Parenting is going to require a lot of you, and some themes start to emerge in the throes of parenthood: love, responsiveness, and demandingness. Being aware of these themes will help you understand how you should begin to respond to the baby after they arrive.

Themes of Parenting

Love is an overwhelming feeling of warmth and connection toward another human being or really any other being. Some new parents don't feel this love right away for an infant. This isn't a red flag by itself, and parents who don't feel a love at first sight sensation for their infants are not bad parents. Newborns offer very little in the way of loving affirmations. They don't tell you anything about how they are feeling, and at times you may wonder if they even know you are there or if they like you. (Note: You are their everything; they do know you are there; they more than like you, they *need* you.) It is ok to take time to learn how to love and nurture your baby. Again, no one will question the depth of this love … no one that is, except maybe you? Particularly for birth parents, the immediate postpartum period is fraught with recovery, an altered body, and hormonal mayhem. Understanding that love might not materialize right away is important to help with your mental health and help you cope with the major life event you just experienced. Mustering up the endless and expansive love you dreamed of for the new human in your care can be exhausting right after delivery; let it be a lifelong pursuit. It's ok to not feel like the relationship with your newborn is the best you've ever had right off the bat. It's hard when you don't know someone but feel you should want to love them more than anyone else in the world. Before you even meet, give yourself the grace and time to allow your love to grow. When I was pregnant with my first baby, I wasn't sure I made the right decision. I was sick, tired, and grappling with not feeling like myself. How did I want this so badly, yet was handling the whole pregnancy process so poorly? I had to take moments out of my day to think about the baby, about how much I wanted this new relationship, about family and what that meant to me. I didn't love every minute of being pregnant, and I knew I wouldn't love every minute of being a new mom, but I wanted my love for my baby to grow to become deeply powerful and expansive. And I let my dream of that kind of love help me get through the hard parts of achieving it. If you are one of the lucky ones who find love immediately upon arrival of your baby, be prepared to bottle those feelings for the times when parenting makes a lot less emotional sense. The only thing you can really be certain of is that you will feel differently after delivery, and not feeling completely in love all the time is perfectly human.

Responsiveness is your ability and willingness to respond to changing needs, and the needs of infants are all over the place. Infants need you to respond to them but don't tell you how to respond or what they need when they want you. Crying is the one way they know how to get you to care for them. The cry works well; it's a sound that can make any parent buckle. Crying is not pleasant, so parents may get the perception they are doing everything wrong. In time, cries can be deciphered, and what a baby wants can be recognized. Know this before the baby comes, so when they scream at you and you feel like you're being punched in the gut, you also leave space for understanding and trying to learn why they are calling to you. Ultimately, what the baby really *needs* is for you to care about them and address them—even if you aren't sure what problem you are trying to solve. Literally, just someone who cares, even if they aren't overcome by love at first sight and don't have all the answers right away. An infant feels secure by having someone there for them. Your infant needs you to respond to them, attempt to understand them, and be able to adapt (just like they are) to a changed world. Being there, responding, holding, talking, laughing, crying, and carrying a baby represent a high level of responsive parenting and fill the newborn's need for connection and a capable presence. Of note, this doesn't only fall on the birth parent. Having one responsive and loving caregiver is all an infant needs, and that person does not need to be you all the time. It can be their second mom, a father, a grandparent, a babysitter, a nanny, a grandparent, a sister, an uncle— another adult who can jump in and respond calmly to their growing needs. Think about the most responsive and committed people in your life and make them a part of getting to know who your baby is.

Demandingness in parenthood is a game of expectations and rule setting. It is much easier to understand the demands of an older child. As kids grow, they talk to you, they want ice cream, they want a new toy truck, they want to watch television. As a parent, you can't give a child everything they want; they must know there are boundaries. Kids learn that you have expectations regarding the things they need to do to achieve their goals and limits to what can be achieved. If they want a new toy, for instance, they need to help their parent with chores around the house. A demanding baby is different. They don't tell you what they want or need, and they don't follow rules or expectations. For unstructured families, this might be exhilarating! No rules! But, remember, babies are individuals with their own free will and commonly a set temperament. Even if you logically know you can't make a baby do anything, you may still have expectations about how you want them to act. For example, you may want your baby to sleep through the night at 6 weeks. I mean, that's what your first baby did, so won't this one do the same thing? But your baby doesn't understand your expectations, and their bodies might not be able to follow your rules. No two babies are alike, and newborns can truly change every day; that's the only rule to embrace or expect about their behavior.

This is where the demandingness of newborn parenting comes in and what you should think about before having a baby. *You* need to set boundaries for how *you* will react and care for yourself when you have an infant who needs someone all the time. The demandingness of newborn parenting really comes from having to be vigilant and make every single decision for them without input or recognition of your new cognitive burden. Decision fatigue and the constant responsiveness you are required to muster to keep up with their incredible development are exhausting. The whole experience demands! Know your limits, set them for yourself, but don't expect your baby to be aware of them or help you dictate the self-care you need. Parenting demands from you an entirely new level of self-insight.

Adjusting Expectations While You're Expecting

So how do you become a loving, responsive parent who understands your baby's demands but is still flexible and fun? You can start before the baby arrives. Be honest about what you envision for a life with a newborn. Do you think it will be fun to hang out and watch trashy reality television 24/7? Are you expecting to have time to take up crocheting, and be able to handcraft a ton of seasonal baby bonnets for your new little one? Maybe you've already had a baby, and it was overwhelming because every time you took a shower, they cried so you never felt you could properly clean. It's ok to want things to go a certain way with your baby. It's great to think about how you might interact and bond before the baby arrives. Let yourself dream about life with a new baby, but don't think that every expectation you have will become a reality. Remember, you have no idea who this person is.

The first few weeks of living with a baby are about giving yourself time to learn what your newborn is *actually* like. With a newborn, the most active form of listening is observation. Many babies will show you their temperament in the first few weeks after birth. Their personality (ie, the combination of things that make up their character) can change as they grow and learn, but their underlying temperament is hardwired. Start to observe your baby for who they will be as they get older. Make doing so a priority. Be mindful about building time into your day to just watch your baby be themselves. When they are awake, what pushes them to cry? What makes them fall asleep? What wakes them up? Do they have different types of cries you can start to make out? Whom do they attach to when held, and whom do they seem uncomfortable with? Start to just notice things about your baby, and don't try to change them—infants don't really understand rules and boundaries. (For more information see "Getting to Know Baby While Taking Care of Yourself" later in this chapter.) Instead, consider the guidelines and guardrails you are going to put in place for yourself as a parent and a person to be able to care for this demanding creature. Prepare to be passive, and look for ways to listen.

My expectations for my first baby were that I was going to be so into it and on top of my baby's needs. I was a trained pediatrician, did extra training to care for babies, and felt like I understood them. I thought my baby would cry, I'd find the problem, fix it, and then no worries! This was definitely *my problem* in retrospect because my daughter was a crier, and sometimes nothing I did made a difference. In hindsight, I think she might have been diagnosed with colic had I shared more with my pediatrician. I expected to be a baby whisperer, and it hurt me when she cried, in part because I was not. I had to learn that my first daughter was hypersensitive to certain sounds and positions. I had to practice walking around the house with her with a hand on her belly or throw her over my shoulder because this was her preferred mode of transport. She is a classic introvert who is slow to warm but loyal and caring when she knows someone well. She wasn't going to engage with me or anyone else unless she felt comfortable doing so. My ever-willing, smiling, extroverted second baby was different. He loved any position I held him in, and we both got energy from crowds and loved to be surrounded by people. Did I parent them differently as newborns to make one inward looking and the other a total extrovert? The short answer is no. They have very different temperaments, and that affects how I parent them as they grow. They show me more of who they are every day. But from day 1, some of the fundamental aspects of their personalities were already there. I just had to look, listen, and adjust my responses and parenting style accordingly.

Getting to Know My Baby

I am saying you need to literally observe and listen to your baby. Ask yourself why they have certain reactions to different situations and people and let that be your day. If only we were all incredibly active listeners or observers—I'm still developing those skills into my 40s. So do you have to spend every second of every day just staring at this baby? No, you would go insane. To do this well, you are going to ask other trusted adults to help you. Especially if you are the birth parent who needs time to recover after delivery. You should never be a lone wolf watching over baby—even wolves travel in packs. Think of who your trusted adults are and be ready to call on them when it's right for your family. Some birth parents like having the grandparents with them right after delivery; they don't find that stressful. Some parents just want the nuclear family to be together for a week or so before inviting others to come and help out. Some families just have a single parent, and so it's important to find support groups or outside help (eg, friends, cousins, babysitters) to build in times when you aren't constantly looking after the baby. Remember, whatever plan you make can be changed after the baby arrives, so alert your support people they will need to be flexible. You will know what you need after you meet the baby, and it can be challenging to figure it all out beforehand. But identifying who can be there to support you, and being able to ask for that support, is a key part of parenting.

Now, let's think of some ways to balance your needs in your relationship with your infant against their needs as newborns. Again, you can't know exactly how you will act until you have the baby in hand, carrier, or bassinet—no one can tell you the type of relationship you are about to build when they don't know you or your infant. You can think of how you will modulate your responses to a needy little one and consider your needs when cultivating this relationship. Parents often report that their wishes and desires get sidelined with a newborn. I always tell families this: Healthy parent = healthy baby. The things you say and do matter; *you matter*.

You already know or have heard about the things that will be fun or maybe challenging about having a newborn. (See "Getting to Know Baby While Taking Care of Yourself" later in this chapter.) You might have had a baby already. That said, it's important to envision how you can address each of your infants as individuals, or what you might do differently to avoid getting frustrated by things that can make parenting overwhelming the first time around. It is a lot to carry a newborn, to feel the amazing joy of having one, and to experience the exhausting reality of being your baby's number 1 for hopefully the rest of their lives!

Getting to Know Baby While Taking Care of Yourself

	PARENT/ CAREGIVER NEEDS	NEWBORN NEEDS	MEETING EVERYONE'S NEEDS
Sleep	Adults need about 8 hours of sleep in 24 hours. Recognition of circadian (day/night) rhythms Tools to cope with sleep deprivation	Infants need about 18 hours of sleep in 24 hours. No day/night differentiation until **around** age 6 months (for some infants it can be slightly shorter, for others it may take a year or more to establish circadian rhythms) A safe sleep environment	Plan nighttime supports: Breastfeeding but passing infant to another caregiver for diaper changes/ swaddling Planning who will perform and help with feeds overnight Being ok with not getting your normal daily tasks done and prioritizing rest (What does your 60% of full capacity look like? Your 80%?) Making time for naps (not when the baby sleeps—let's just call that advice bananas); when you actually feel tired, who can take over?
Exercise	20 minutes of moderate-intensity physical activity every day Make 2 of your days strength activities, and the rest cardio. Immune system and **mental health** (!!!) benefits—this is not exercise to return your body to its prepregnancy form; it's to keep your mind healthy no matter your weight. Ditch your scale.	Being moved into different positions when held, fed, or placed in crib To view some examples of breast-feeding positions you can check here: To view some examples of tummy time you can check here: 	Having your infant next to you during workout sessions on a flat, hard surface (in bassinet, on a blanket on the floor) Recruiting another caregiver so you can get your 20 minutes of exercise in Being ok with not getting your 20 minutes, but making some space for movement that works with your schedule (eg, taking your infant for a walk outside)

	PARENT/ CAREGIVER NEEDS	NEWBORN NEEDS	MEETING EVERYONE'S NEEDS
Socialization	Improves mental health Helps with motivation Gives space for talking about and debriefing on parenting	One consistent, responsive, and loving caregiver at all times Early literacy to boost brain health and development (Read to your baby often.) Limited exposure to crowds	Time with another parent/caregiver/adult built into the day Recruiting babysitters, friends, relatives, or others to help out Online supports, including parenting groups, chats, virtual meetings Community supports, including local baby groups
Recognition	Desire to know you are parenting well Remembering that being a parent is only a part of who you are Remaining connected with core values and beliefs	A baby never needs alone time; they need a loving caregiver around at all times. Periods of minimal stimulation or quiet awake time	Before you deliver, write notes to yourself as reminders of what you are taking on and how to give yourself grace. Reaching into your social networks for support after delivery Having discussions with pediatricians or other medical professionals when you are feeling low

Infant Parenting: A Small Space

There are many different types of self-proclaimed parenting styles. But you are not just one parenting style; you and your infant are unique and the whole experience of parenting is dynamic. Parenting will take many forms as your baby grows, but the core foundation of parenting well is your adaptability and flexibility. Especially when that child is an infant. You want to be a loving and responsive parent, and you want to be sensitive to the new rhythms and stages your child will face.

A responsive parent understands that their needs and their infant's needs are different and works to reconcile those differences in a way that will keep each individual cared for. Responsive parenting means not thinking the baby can behave better, or that it's the newborn's job to learn to be on their schedule or respond to their prompting in a certain way. A baby will let you how they feel and give you a sense of their temperament, but that's about it. Parenting a newborn requires adapting to their needs and creating space for them, a skill that can be learned. A responsive parent isn't happy or easygoing all the time; no one is. A responsive parent can calmly observe their infant crying in one moment, and then leave the room and scream into a pillow in the next. It is ok to become frustrated or upset if you are not jiving with your baby. Right after birth, most parents have low emotional reserves because so much of their home life has changed. Having a new person around and getting to know them is hard work. Parents feel excited, tired, happy, stressed—a melting pot of complex and intense emotions centering around the fact that a family structure is forever altered. You have brought a new person into the mix, one who is really relying on you. You have to ditch your expectations and learn about this person and how you can parent them, love them, and still feel like yourself. It's a lot to take in, and it's not going to be easy right off the bat. Adjusting will take time.

That's why it's ok to have complex feelings about caring for an infant. Most people do. It means you care about how your life is changing. You are forging a relationship with a person who can give you little feedback, and is unaware of the boundaries they are pushing and the intense care they need. Listen to the baby and yourself, talk to others, and find community with family, support groups of other new parents, or people in virtual spaces. Take things one day at a time and don't try to be the best or the most or the *[insert your own superlative of greatness here]*. Sometimes being a responsive parent means surviving in the moment. If your feelings are outside of what you think is typical for a parent, don't be afraid to talk about it. Get help to manage your changing body, identity, and home life. We will go over who to talk to and where to get help in a later chapter. Just remember, you are going to be doing a lot. This requires a shift in perspective.

With the demandingness, frustration, and joy that can accompany infant care, the actual world for you and baby is *very small*. You will soon be watching a small human who mostly sleeps, and trying to learn who they are, all in the space of your living quarters day in and day out. This is a shrinking space for some families—and that might be great! Maybe the only place on Earth you want to be is in a room with your newborn. Others might feel as if they are slowly sinking into a couch cushion (hopefully, your living room or den has one comfy couch on which to sit through the weight of infant care) and are losing touch with some aspects of life. Always go back to your purpose or drive in taking care of a newborn. Why did you want this person in your family? What do you hope they will bring? How do you envision responding to the newborn in front of you? Recognize that the newborn period looks and feels different for everyone, and your relationship with baby will be different from any other you have had.

TIPS FOR PARENTING BEFORE MEETING BABY

Recognize the importance of attachment: This is the most important human need.

Think of trusted individuals you want in your baby's life, and recruit them to be a part of it.

Give yourself time to heal if you are the birth parent.

Think of your expectations about parenting a newborn or what you are worried about. Realize these are your thoughts and aren't necessarily what baby will do.

Understand that your baby is born with a temperament, and although their personality is evolving, this temperament may be hardwired.

Be ready to actively listen to and observe your newborn.

Wonder about the person you are going to raise and who you want them to be.

Practice adaptability and flexibility—if your expectations aren't met, will you cry? Need a break? What are your must-dos to parent well, and what can you let go of?

Now on to your delivery. Let's meet this baby.

Chapter 2

A Delivery

*M*y hospital pager (that's right, pager, and yes I know technology is better than this now) went off in the late afternoon. "Failure to progress, nonreassuring fetal heart tracing, peds to delivery." As a neonatologist and the only baby doctor in the hospital that day, I am peds—short for pediatrics–so I made my way downstairs to labor and delivery from the neonatal intensive care unit (NICU). Walking into the labor room, I found my team—a neonatal nurse practitioner, respiratory therapist, and neonatal nurse—assembling at the infant's bedside checking equipment and awaiting our patient. I asked one of the labor and delivery nurses for the full scoop. "She has been pushing for 4 hours. They offered her a cesarean section (c-section) because she had been pushing for so long and the baby's tracing (that's medical speak for heart rate) doesn't always look good, but she declined and really wants a vaginal delivery, so here we are." I nodded. The birth parent was screaming; she hadn't had an epidural and the pain seemed to be excruciating. I settled into the room with my team and just waited. As she was pushing, the patient started to describe the pain as burning, and the obstetrician mentioned something called the "ring of fire." This is when the infant's head is crowning or coming out of the vaginal opening and it burns, burns, burns: the ring of fire. Having not yet had any children, I asked my team if they had experienced this; all had heard of it. The neonatal nurse practitioner then started mumbling the lyrics to "I Walk the Line" as we waited for the baby to make their way through the "line."

*After a few long minutes, the baby came out in the occiput pos-
terior position or "sunny side up." Delicious when ordering eggs, but
not when referring to a delivery. In most deliveries, the infant's face is
toward the birth parent's back. In the occiput posterior position, the
face is toward the stomach and gets pressed up against the pelvic bone.
Many times, the infant's face gets bruised, and the birth parent's body
gets torn. This baby came out blue, limp, and lifeless. I could feel my
muscles tensing, and immediately my team went to work to hear the
baby cry. We like to hear a baby's cry. We usually start by stimulating
and then suctioning any blood and amniotic fluid from the mouth.
We then put a mask over the newborn's nose and mouth to breath
for them if they won't do it themselves. This baby only needed a little
encouragement, though, and the cry came and my shoulders relaxed.
The birth parent was exhausted, her body had suffered a fourth-degree
laceration where the vaginal tissue gets ripped through all the way
to the anus. It was going to be a long repair for the obstetricians. The
nonbirth parent came over to see the baby, timidly touching them after
their dramatic entrance through the ring of fire. "What's the baby's
name?" I asked. He smiled. "Cash." My nurse practitioner gently hip
checked me and I smiled. "That's funny," I said. "I was sure it would
be Johnny."*

Expectant parents often put a lot of thought and energy into
their mode of delivery and the immediate hours and days after it
occurs. There is pressure on parents to think that the only "natural" delivery is a vaginal birth. And a belief that a deviation from
their birth plan is a surrender of their hopes and dreams for their
life-changing event.

No matter how your baby enters the world, what's *really* important
is making time and space to meet and get to know your baby. If I,
as a neonatologist, were to make a birth plan, it would read something like:

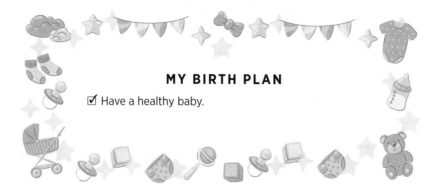

MY BIRTH PLAN

☑ Have a healthy baby.

What's in an Actual Birth Plan?

Many birth plans are much more detailed than this. Let's break down an example of a birth plan and discuss what's in them. And why I'm not against them and why I don't think you should hold yourself to one. A birth plan is a written document that you have or that lives in your medical record and lays out your preferences for your delivery.

This type of plan can also include things like

- The name and phone number of your doctor
- Medications you want during delivery like an epidural
- The equipment you might need
- Names of your support people during the birth
- Your wishes for feeding, rest, and medical interventions for the baby

Some new parents find so much joy in creating their birth plans—the ability to envision how a very important life event will go. You want to dream about it and get excited about it despite the fact you know it will be painful in the moment. Some people also need to gain knowledge as a means of coping with a big life event. Others might want to follow their plan exactly because they need to feel they are in control during an experience that's hard to predict or anticipate.

SAMPLE BIRTH PLAN

Labor

☐ I would like to move around.

☐ I would like to drink fluids.

Anesthesia

☐ I want to discuss options with the doctor.

☐ I want a natural birth.

I prefer

☐ An intravenous (IV) line for fluids and medications

☐ A heparin or saline locked IV so I have access but am not hooked up to anything

I want the following people with me (list here):

_____

_____

_____

It is ok, or it is not ok to have medical trainees (medical students, residents) in my delivery.

If available, I would like

☐ A birthing ball

☐ A birthing stool

☐ A birthing chair

☐ A squat bar

☐ A warm shower or bath (Note: a bath can only be given in the first stage of labor.)

Baby

☐ I would like to breastfeed immediately after delivery.

☐ I would like to talk to a breastfeeding consultant.

This is what is so great about having a plan; you can start to understand, gain information, and think about the moment of delivery.

I wish I could describe the intense satisfaction I experience when I create and execute a checklist. When I make a to-do list, it is with the express purpose of meeting every item on it. I am also a doctor so, yes, I am more likely than most to exhibit signs of obsessive-compulsive disorder. When making a check mark with my hand, there is something so sweet about the sharp turn downward and then the effortless letting go of the right side of the check mark. It's like meditation, a release! If I had a plan that I wasn't able to follow, my hands would be shaking. I'd be pretty upset because I would have put *a lot* of thought into my plan, and I'd want to follow it perfectly. Sure, they tell you it might not go how you want during your delivery, but you hope that it will. You start to ground yourself in the use of a certain amount of oxytocin. Or the fact that you won't need pain medication at all. And not being able to follow your meticulously researched plan might feel like a derailment. Dealing with the unexpected when you're expecting is hard. Having a baby is such a big deal.

This gets to the potential downsides of a very detailed birth plan. Because while you know that things might not go exactly as you planned, the ways in which your baby's birth occurs can go in directions you might never have envisioned. I think there is this perception that physicians don't like birth plans because of the issue of control. I have heard patients talk about how their doctors don't want them dictating their exact delivery plan, and thus feel like their doctors don't care about their experience. This is *not* true. Doctors want what is best for the birth parent and the baby in a delivery. The only reason I don't want someone attached to a care plan is that it doesn't leave room for the twists and turns of birth, delivery, and raising a child. It is so hard for humans to watch other humans experience disappointment and defeat in the face of something no one can truly predict. This is an event that is supposed to be joyful but at times can be filled with unanticipated challenges. To see families become

despondent and desperate to follow a plan they were attached to and
see scribbles on a page instead of check marks is hard for everyone. Remember, your medical team genuinely wants you to have a
healthy, safe, and happy delivery. And your pediatrician wants to
prepare you to parent in a digital age in which information is abundant, expectations are high, and the unexpected is hard to face when
there is so much information on hand.

To illustrate how delivery and parenting have changed, let's compare it to the weather. Every morning when I wake up, I obsessively
think about it, then scroll through my weather app on my phone. The
thought of going outside not fully prepared for hail or without my
sunglasses on a bright and cheerful day makes me anxious. Having a
newborn is in so many ways similar to not having a weather app, or
24/7 access to radar so you can watch how the clouds move across the
sky. When you walk through the door of a hospital for your delivery (and into the realm of parenting), you have to come prepared to
weather anything. We are talking about an emotional suitcase full of
clothes for every climate, a parka stuffed next to swimwear. You are
going to have to mentally prepare yourself to step outside, take in the
temperature, and plan based on what you see as opposed to what you
want or are hoping your day will be like. I've seen families who've had
uneventful deliveries with healthy babies get really upset about an
extra fluid bolus they received, or their newborn's having had routine
testing performed without their express consent—that is, routine
testing for something the hospital doesn't even have a consent form
for. It clouds the joyous time they could be having with their new little
human, igniting frustration and anxiety instead of opening the door to
see if it's really raining or is a perfectly sunny day. I'm writing this book
on parenting a newborn for you, but it's really just to say that parenting
doesn't come with plans or guidebooks. It comes with love, hopes, and
dreams. Rather than hoping to have the perfect sunny birth, anchoring
yourself in the emotions you may feel for your baby in the moment is a

more fulfilling way to use your time and energy. A delivery may take a few hours or days, but it's the moments after birth when the hands-on baby bonding begins.

Consider a Vision Board, Not a Birth Plan

Instead of making a birth plan (but believe me, we will talk about birth in a second…), I challenge you to make a vision board for yourself. Not for your baby, but for how you envision your relationship with that person.

How to Make a Vision Board

- Give yourself a few hours (about 3 to 5, perhaps an entire afternoon).
- Get creative with supplies for your project: poster board, cork board, white board, construction paper, photos, magazine cutouts, markers, etc.
- Thinking about what it means to be a successful parent and have a thriving relationship with your baby, consider these 4 categories for your vision board:
  - **Happiness**—What will bring you joy as a parent? What about an infant who will bring you joy? Are there people you want to share this experience with?
  - **Achievement**—What do you hope to accomplish as a parent? What would make you feel the most successful as a parent? Is getting 6 hours of sleep no matter what the most important thing to you?
  - **Significance**—How will you record your journey through parenting? What moments will you look back on? What experiences will be most meaningful for baby and for you?
  - **Legacy**—What traits do you hope to pass down to your child?

- Divide your board, use your supplies, make it pretty.
- Display your work in a place that will remind you not to get bogged down by the moment but will allow you to experience the entirety of what you are creating.

Sample Vision Board, Made During My Third Pregnancy

I still have this vision board on my kitchen wall. When I'm walking around with the baby I look at it and am reminded of the things I want for her. It's prompted me to read her a book or snap an extra photo of her. It motivates me to express my love for her, so I don't know if I'll ever take it down.

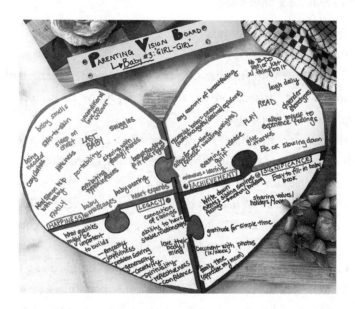

Two Ways Out: Venerated Vaginal Births and Surgical C-Sections

For context, the births I attend professionally are essentially always at risk for diverting from expectations—both those of the doctors and those of the parents. I knew going into my own hospital birth that

I didn't have full control over the mode of my delivery. I wanted a vaginal delivery, like many parents, but if a c-section was recommended to help give the baby and me a healthy start, I was going to take it. Would I be disappointed if I had one? Absolutely. Would that affect my relationship with my infant? Yes, I'd be sad. The recovery I anticipated would be different and relationship-building with my newborn would be different. But forming new relationships means learning to manage the uncertainty that comes with them.

Most parents are well-versed in the 2 options for delivery: the often-exalted vaginal birth and the surgical c-section. What you might not know is that for the past several years there has been an increase in the number of c-section deliveries. Physicians, scientists, and physician-scientists (the combination does exist) can't exactly explain why, and they hate not knowing. It seems to be due to a variety of factors, including age of the parents, their body habits, how the baby is positioned inside, whether they're having multiple babies, and parental preference, to name just a few reasons. With this rise in c-sections has come the promotion and support of vaginal deliveries, which can offer advantages for the parent and baby. It has also led to a rise in the casual villainization of c-sections as an undesired mode of delivery. This is not the case for the parents and babies who have, want, or need them.

Medical professionals have tried to address the rising c-section rate in part because there are benefits to babies when a vaginal delivery is possible. When born vaginally, newborns often experience the wonders of labor (birth parents will argue about the wonder part). Labor is more than just painful (though boy is it painful). It's also instructive. It helps babies become a little bit stressed and produce hormones called catecholamines (think steroids) to get them amped up to enter the world. These catecholamines jump-start blood flow to the brain and heart, and get the lungs prepared to breathe air. With some c-sections, infants don't get the benefits of performance-enhancing hormones prior to their debut. This makes them more likely to visit me in the NICU, particularly for breathing issues.

So how does your delivery factor into the critical relationship you are forming with your infant? Early on, it can have a major influence on your recovery and on your emotions. Often, it is more difficult to bounce back from a c-section than from a vaginal delivery. Cutting through abdominal muscle limits the amount of movement and the amount of weight a mom can carry. It can also make birth parents prone to infection and scarring. But if you remember the Johnny Cash story at the beginning of this chapter, vaginal deliveries are not without a recovery period or without discomfort to the baby. The issues are just *different*. Infants can get stuck in the vaginal canal and require assistance to get out. Birth parents can face tears in the vaginal wall and beyond, have bleeding, and suffer incontinence or pelvic floor dysfunction—meaning the muscles of the pelvic floor aren't as strong or are strained (think peeing every time you sneeze).

In the end, not having the delivery you planned for might be a reality. But, hopefully, it was a healthy and safe option for you and your baby. It doesn't mean you've failed at childbirth or are a bad parent. Delivery is not like taking a final exam in a college biology course. Your body receives an A+ just by getting through it. Remember, no matter your mode of delivery, the only thing you should assign value to in the birth experience is keeping you and the baby healthy and safe so your relationship in the outside world can begin.

Hang-ups With Home Births

Where should this glorious new relationship with your baby begin? The fourth floor of hospital building C sounds perfect. Does this hospital take reservations? I want it to be quiet so we can talk and bond together ASAP.

Some families try to decide between meeting their baby at home, at a birthing center, or at a hospital. To my knowledge, no one has ever surveyed neonatologists in the United States about where they deliver their babies. I bet if you asked, nearly 100% of us have delivered in a hospital. One neonatology friend told me she wanted to be at a hospital that could place her baby on a heart and lung machine "just in case." That's extreme, but being knowledgeable about the medical capacities at the hospital isn't. After birth, literally every minute counts for a baby who needs help. That is why we have something called the Apgar score in medicine. A mnemonic device for the Apgar score is *a*ppearance (pink or blue? I'm talking skin color here), *p*ulse (heart rate), *g*rimace (they all look a little grumpy about leaving the womb), *a*ctivity (moving of their arms and legs), and *r*espirations (breathing). It's named after Dr Virginia Apgar, who created the score to help assess how babies enter the world. The Apgar score is given at 1 minute and 5 minutes after birth—that's how much time you often have to help a baby breathe—just 5 minutes. Neonatologists know this and are trained in how to react quickly in a delivery room when a baby needs us. Not all hospitals have neonatologists, though, so here are some questions to ask about the baby care in the hospital where you deliver.

Questions About Supports for Baby in Hospital

- Are there neonatologists or pediatricians who help deliver babies?
- Is the staff trained in neonatal resuscitation?
- Is there a NICU at this hospital? What types of babies do they care for?
- Would my baby need to be transferred to a larger children's hospital if they were not doing well after delivery? Which one would it be?

There are many anecdotes about the joys of home birth. Data does show there seem to be some better birth parent outcomes with a home birth. If you deliver at home, there is generally less instrumentation of your vagina and less use of things like forceps and vacuums to assist in the delivery. So maybe your recovery will be better? Or maybe not. We don't have great information about that. That said, it is nice to be in a familiar and comfortable place.

However, a home birth also means there is less monitoring of the baby and you. If something goes amiss, you might not realize it right away. You'd have more interventions in a hospital setting because if there is cause for worry, there are more ways to address that worry and help you and baby. Health care professionals tend to be conservative (maybe that's why c-sections are increasing?). We've seen and treated a lot of birth parents and newborns, which means unexpected outcomes at deliveries are expected. We are able to head off a problem if we suspect it's coming.

Hospital protocols are meant to keep you safe. A nurse checking your blood pressure at 3:00 am can be intrusive, but it's also protective of your health. The truth about delivery in the United States is that the risks of childbirth are high, even today. So, yes, you give up some control and comfort delivering in the hospital, but the tradeoff is safety. If a baby needs help, the baby will get help fast.

Most newborns respond well to resuscitative efforts. Stimulating and suctioning Cash (in the earlier example) got him to cry right away. But if a baby does not have access to skilled professionals who can intervene, they could need more help when you do get to a hospital. Imagine it's just you, a scared partner, and a birth attendant; this can lead to an immensely stressful first meeting with the baby. If you want the experience to be one in which a new life enters yours and relationship building begins in earnest, your best bet is to do that in a place that respects and understands what a feat childbirth is. That place is not in your living room. It's having access to a hospital room in a birthing center or a hospital. This is especially true in the United States where we don't have streamlined or centralized health care, and access differs a lot depending on where you live. That is why the American Academy of Pediatrics recommends against home births; they can be dangerous to the baby and we want your meeting them to be nothing but joyous. This can make getting to a hospital in an emergency difficult in and of itself.

Delivering at home in other countries, such as some European countries, results in slightly better outcomes for babies. But even in European countries there are reports of slightly worse outcomes for infants born at home, or no difference between home and the hospital. So overall, hospitals are just the safest places to deliver. Efforts are underway to make home births more accessible and safe for families, especially those who feel discriminated against when they enter a hospital. I'm hopeful that home births may become a much better and safer option for families in the future. If you are seriously considering one, talk to your doctor so you are not making this decision on your own. Doctors generally use the following criteria (and others) in the table titled "Planned Home Birth Considerations" to help families with this choice.

PLANNED HOME BIRTH CONSIDERATIONS

- No known diseases or pregnancy complications

- Baby is 37 to 41 weeks at the time of delivery

- It's just 1 baby

- Baby is in a head-down position

- Labor that is spontaneous or induced as an outpatient

Have supports in place

- A physician or a midwife certified by the American Midwifery Certification Board or whose education and licensure meet the International Confederation of Midwives Global Standards for Midwifery Education

Practices within an integrated and regulated health system

- Attendance by at least 2 care providers, one who is trained and responsible for the care of the newborn

- Availability of appropriate equipment for the baby

- Ready access to medical consultation

- Access to safe and timely transport to a nearby hospital with a preexisting arrangement

Adapted with permission from *Pediatrics*. 2020;146(3):e2020015511.

No matter how or where you deliver your newborn, you are going to become a new parent. So think about that moment right after you deliver your baby and you look into their eyes. How you want to build that emotional connection, and learn to trust each other and your parenting.

Chapter 3

Your Placental Relationship

*O*ne day I saw a family eating the placenta at their baby's bedside in the neonatal intensive care unit (NICU). It was blended with other ingredients and closely resembled a strawberry-banana smoothie. I could see pieces of it entering the birth parent's mouth as they sipped with a long opaque straw. Our befuddled care team was in a tizzy for 2 reasons. The first and most pressing was that hospitals must follow strict infection protocols, and eating a placenta at the bedside seemed like it might violate one of them. In general, NICUs don't allow food and drink to be consumed in patient care areas, but no one could rightly say if a placenta counted as an actual food or a drink. The second reason was we lacked an understanding of why someone would eat a placenta. Regrettably, I didn't get the chance to interview this family about their "placentophagy" (the fancy term coined for eating your placenta). They finished the smoothie well before I got a chance to try to convince them not to.

A Fleeting Organ

Baby comes out, and the placenta is not far behind. If you are struggling with what to do with your placenta, stop now. The afterbirth should be an afterthought. Attaching yourself or your baby to the placenta isn't helping to facilitate your growing relationship. In fact, I've seen the placenta be a hinderance to bonding with the baby. Any energy spent fretting about how you will care for, season, or prepare a placenta will take time away from focusing on the baby.

Does this mean the placenta is trash? Of course not. The placenta is a complex and beautiful bag of blood, etched with interwoven parental and baby blood vessels in small spirals and intricate turns. It is a powerhouse, forming with the growing fetus and responsible for the baby's growth inside the birth parent. If the placenta can't support the baby, there is no other organ that offers to step in and help. Thanks a lot colon!

The placenta begins to develop when a bunch of cells that developed from a fertilized egg make their way to the uterine wall—usually at around week 2 of a pregnancy. Those cells start to dig into the wall, and eventually alter the blood supply from the uterus and create the placenta. The powers of the placenta include transfer of nutrients and antibodies made by the birth parent to help prevent infection and acting as a baby's heart and lungs. Placental issues can be a cause of poor growth of the fetus in the womb, infections, and preterm birth. Neonatologists are often curious to see or hear about placentas after delivery when caring for a sick or small baby. The placenta can give us clues regarding the best way to treat our tiny patients. For example, I've seen placentas in which the blood vessels didn't form properly so the fetus didn't get the oxygen and blood it needed to develop. Or placentas that contained a lot of inflammation, indicating they were fighting an infection or some other process was occurring with the immune system that made the placenta unhappy.

Even for a healthy placenta, though, we don't know exactly what triggers a birth parent to go into labor; however, we think the placenta's slowly dying could be the start of the process. The poetry of one of the most fleeting organs. As the pregnancy gets close to 40 weeks, the placenta begins to calcify and lose its nutrient-giving powers. After 40 weeks, neonatologists say nothing good happens inside for the baby. While all neonatologists respect and revere the majestic placenta, after it grows a baby—or multiple babies, as sometimes they can share a placenta—it's done. It becomes inefficient and its powers rapidly dwindle. Babies reach a point at which they are better off receiving nutrients from milk than from blood, and birth occurs.

After a baby is born, the placenta—also called the afterbirth—must follow. A birth parent must push out the tissue that helped support the fetus. In my third pregnancy, I had an accessory placenta, meaning a tiny piece of placenta was separate from the larger body of the organ. In these situations they had to check my uterus with an ultrasound after I delivered to make sure all the placenta was out. Any placenta left inside the body is at risk of causing infection or a lot of bleeding. Because the placenta is a hormonal mess, like we can be after delivery, birth parents with retained placenta (that is, placenta that is still inside them) can have issues with the milk supply when they are breastfeeding. So, getting out the whole placenta is key. Luckily, this is not as painful as pushing out a baby, as the placenta is a wet soggy sack. If it doesn't all come out, the best time to find it is right after your cervix is open after delivery, so your doctor might get really handsy if there is any worry the placenta could still be lodged inside you.

All that said, the placenta is not an organ you need to bond with—you only need a baby to bond with.

Cutting the Cord

While cutting a baby's nails gives me palpitations (yes, I've made my baby's poor finger bleed a little and cried over it), cutting a baby's umbilical cord makes sense. I've had to counsel some families that want to do what is termed a *lotus birth* or more formally *umbilical nonseverance*. This is a practice in which the placenta is left attached until it falls off "naturally." This can take up to 2 weeks. Why would families want to do this? It is a spiritual practice for some, though, to my knowledge, no formal organized religion endorses this activity. Understanding the umbilical cord will help explain why this practice has gained some popularity despite a lack of scientific evidence to support it.

The anatomy of the umbilical cord is simple: a little bit of jelly (named after Wharton, a British physician) and blood vessels— usually 2 arteries and 1 vein. The main function of the umbilical cord is to deliver nutrient-rich blood from the placenta to the fetus. Given that it has blood coursing through it, if one were to cut it immediately after birth, things would get messy. Think blood coming out of a firehose and someone fumbling to clamp it off. If you find yourself in a situation where you are delivering a baby outside of a hospital, tying off the umbilical cord is a must. Any string or shoelace will do.

One practice for which there are some data is delayed umbilical cord clamping. Delayed cord clamping means waiting for at least 1 minute before clamping off or cutting the cord. This is a practice you likely won't even know is happening unless you hear an obstetrician or a pediatrician mention the time. We think delayed clamping is helpful because it gives babies more blood and iron, which, in turn, may help with their brain development. For preterm infants, it has other benefits like reducing the need for blood transfusions, lowering the risk of a certain type of intestinal infection, and decreasing the risks of bleeding in the brain.

This is all good, but even delayed cord clamping can have some potential downsides. In rare cases it increases blood volumes and can lead to polycythemia, which is when the baby experiences complications from having too much blood in their blood vessels, and flow through them is slow and unreliable. Also, more blood can mean higher risk of jaundice, which is in part driven by the breakdown of red blood cells in babies. Jaundice is a yellow skin color that doctors watch for in newborns. (Find more on jaundice in Chapter 5.) That said, the benefits of the practice outweigh the downsides and so we recommend it in almost all deliveries, knowing most babies will tolerate a minute or so of extra blood flow before we cut the cord.

While a delay is ok, you should cut the cord. That's because the risks of leaving a baby attached to a past-prime placenta are higher than any benefit you'd get from leaving it on. In fact, there is no known benefit to a lotus birth or an umbilical nonseverance. If your baby was participating in a study looking into the possible benefits of umbilical nonseverance, that's one thing—and thanks for volunteering in the name of science! But without any proven benefit, in addition to the complexities involved in navigating around the placenta to care for the baby, it's best to just remove it. In all of my deliveries, I worried the umbilical cord would be wrapped around my baby's neck. This does happen sometimes and can make it harder for babies to start breathing when they are born. Luckily, this never happened to me. In fact, in my last delivery, my umbilical cord was extremely short. They couldn't even bring my daughter up past my pelvis because of the teeny tiny cord that held her to the life-giving placenta. I had to have the cord cut so she could come visit me while we waited for my placenta to deliver.

If you don't cut the cord, the alleged benefits of umbilical nonseverance include extra blood volume, the psychological benefit of transitioning into the world with less trauma (because of a cosmic connection between placenta and baby), and maybe a nicer belly button? I've always been fond of outies myself. That said, we know the arteries that pump blood from the placenta to the baby and live in the cord shrivel up and stop beating shortly after the baby is born, so continued blood transfer is unlikely. We also know that infants likely don't remember delivery as their brain isn't well-enough formed to store memories, so a psychological benefit surrounding an added trauma after birth is questionable.

This is what we know for sure. It's natural for bacteria to grow in dark, moist, bloody spaces. If you keep the placenta connected to a baby after birth, it could take 10 or more days to fall off. During this time, the baby might be fine. However, there is the real and reported risk to babies of getting sick from germs multiplying on the raw placental tissue. If you leave the placenta on the baby, you have to care for it. It will start to decompose and smell, so some proponents of this practice encourage parents to rub herbs or salts on the tissue to dry it out. There are no clear practice guidelines on how to do this, and it could be yet another mode of infection. This practice of preserving and perfuming the placenta will take mental energy and time away from getting to know your baby. Additionally, you will need to tuck the placenta into the bassinet and carry it with you. The safe sleep recommendations of the American Academy of Pediatrics stress that nothing is to be in the crib with the baby, like blankets, pillows, or soft toys, and that includes a bagged-up placenta.

Please know that whatever benefits are believed to arise from this practice are not proven. And understand there are other ways to honor the placenta that are less risky to the baby and your relationship with them.

Placenta With a Side of Fries

Let's get back to the placenta smoothie in the NICU. Placentophagy—or eating your placenta—is another practice for which there have been purported benefits, but, again, none are proven. The belief is that you can get iron and hormones from ingesting the placenta, which will accomplish all sorts of wonderful things. Like saving you from postpartum depression or boosting your milk supply if you decide to breastfeed. Truly though, a birthed placenta has already lived its life. Being past its prime, the amount of nutrients it contains is likely minimal.

There are numerous ways to eat a placenta, but this is not a recipe book or a practice I recommend. The most popular way to ingest a placenta is through an encapsulation process in which the parents pay to have the placenta made into palatable swallowable pills. I don't know exactly how this process works, and that's because there is little oversight into how companies manufacture this product. I am often left wondering how many pieces of your placenta are actually in the brown unassuming pellets purported to be postpartum wonders.

Unfortunately, the only thing documented about placentophagy are concerns with regard to infection. Sound familiar? That's because it's the same thing that makes leaving the placenta attached to your baby a potential problem. The Centers for Disease Control and Prevention issued a warning about a particularly nasty bacteria called group B *Streptococcus* (strep) that may have caused infection in a baby whose parent ate the placenta. Was it from the placenta itself or from eating placenta capsules that were contaminated with bacteria? We can't say for sure. However, I will keep coming back to infections as a serious "no go" in the book of neonatology. Neonatologists don't mess with anything that can cause infection in a baby. We have seen too many sick babies fall seriously ill, seemingly within minutes, to not respect how deadly bacteria and viruses can be for our tiniest humans. Infants can't fight infections like adults can, and any pediatrician will tell you that a fever in a newborn is a medical emergency.

Don't do something with your placenta that puts your baby at higher risk of getting sick. Take supplements if you need them; iron and micronutrients are available in many forms. Talk with your doctor about the nutritional supports you need after delivery.

But I don't want you to just leave the placenta in the delivery room if you're going to regret that. Let's get creative about what you can do with your umbilical cord or placenta if you want to keep them.

Artisanal Placentas

I was sad not to have a photo of my first placenta. My husband remembered it and, being squeamish when it comes to blood, almost fainted. Naturally, I had him take a picture of my second placenta, both to test his orthostatic blood pressure and to jog my memories of my second birth. I'm sharing it with you now so I'm not the only one staring longingly at my postpartum memories. (I also have a great shot of my third placenta and it's accessory lobe that I delivered with ease, but I'll spare you the "continued gore").

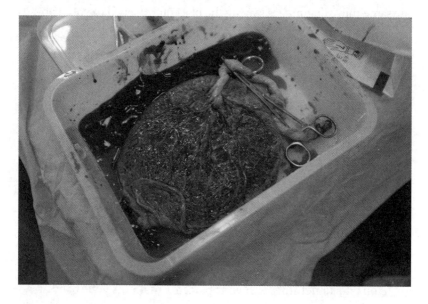

If you are interested in keeping the placenta, by all means do. It will take some organization on your part; ask your doctor about it and see if the hospital will actually let you take it home. Next, after you birthed the baby remind everyone that you want the placenta, or assign your support person the job of keeping track of the placenta. Just make sure you take it off the baby and don't eat it. Find some way to package it, spread it out on a canvas, make a finger paint design or a baby footprint. Let those creative juices go wild. For me, I just wasn't sure where in the house would be the most appropriate place for organ art—maybe the upstairs hallway? I briefly explored placental jewelry. Ultimately though I thought if I got a compliment on my placenta necklace, my knee jerk response would be, "*It's my placenta!*" and that could steal from its beauty and label me as creepy. You can argue I just wasn't creative and cool enough to make room for my placenta outside of a photograph. But if you really want to keep your placenta, make it art!

Cord Keepsakes

If you are like me and physical placental arts and crafts are not your thing, think about saving your cord blood instead. This blood is scientifically miraculous. There are ongoing studies on how to use cord blood as a cure for many diseases. It is a medical therapy with the potential to save lives.

Even after the cord is clamped and stops beating, the magical blood that was pumped to the baby remains in it. The magic really comes from its stem cells. When you hear about stem cells, you probably think they are cells that can become anything. And you're right, they sort of can. Physicians, scientists, and physician-scientists (yes, again a real combo!) are working hard to expand the power of cord blood cells. There is an ever-growing list of medical conditions that could benefit from their use. Should you save your cord blood? The short answer is "yes" definitely; the longer answer is maybe not in the way you think.

I first heard of cord blood banking at the New York City Baby Show, a show geared toward first-time parents. Regretfully, I signed up to get information on the practice of cord blood banking from a *private* bank. I didn't really know how to do it and heard that maybe I should. At the end of the day, signing up for a predatory email list made me more frustrated than educated. I received at least weekly emails and occasional phone calls aggressively encouraging me to buy my way into a cord blood bank. The cost was thousands of dollars up front and yearly storage fees I didn't have. The sales pitch didn't work on an indebted doctor in training.

I'm not going to try and sell you anything. The information I am providing for baby bonding is critical, and the process is inexpensive and easy to do at home. Cord blood banking itself can be *entirely free* when you donate the cord blood to a public bank. Public cord blood banks allow you to donate your cord blood for medical therapies and research, and you aren't charged collection or storage fees. While blood in private banks is only reserved for the people paying for it, blood in public banks is used by society at large. It gets matched to those in need for medical therapies or used for research into different ways to treat people with cord blood. Not a drop goes to waste. Statistically, you are also more likely to need cord blood from a public bank than from a private one. With private banking, there is the possibility that the very disease for which you need treatment lives in your blood, so you can't use the blood you stored to cure yourself or your family. Suffice it to say, public banking winds up being more of a win for you, and with the added benefit of helping a much larger community.

Donating cord blood is a lot like donating regular blood. To donate cord blood you must answer screening questionnaires and be prepared ahead of time, particularly if the hospital at which you deliver your baby doesn't have a seamless way to help arrange the donation. Not all hospitals can support public banking despite the benefit to society, because of all the added resources needed. If you want to publicly bank your cord blood, you should start by telling your obstetrician and finding out if the hospital at which you are planning to deliver accepts these donations. If it doesn't register with a public bank at around 34 weeks. Go through the eligibility screening. Obtain a kit, pack it into your hospital bag, and get ready to ask the hospital staff to help you collect the blood after delivery. Lastly, know that you will be investing in future generations—including your baby's generation—with your actions. For more information on donating cord blood please use this QR code.

You will birth a baby and a placenta, but that's just the start of your journey. An incredible life-changing event ushering in a seminal relationship. The hours or days you spent helping a baby enter the world are nothing compared to what comes after. So many families want to wish away the newborn period because of its unpredictability. But come with me to the shifting reality of newborns and learn to enjoy the ride. Let's get away from placenta plans and start to get into thinking about how you are going to connect and bond with your newborn.

Chapter 4

Let's Get Physical

Working at a teaching hospital can be exhausting. I have had to embrace externalizing the voice inside my head to teach. For a long time, I was awkward about it. Why would this medical student or resident want to know what I was thinking as I was walking, just doing my job? I don't know how many other jobs require you to establish a rapport with families, diagnose and treat conditions in newborns, all while medical students shadow your every move while you try to teach them to do all the things a neonatologist does every day. I need to try and make a lot of people happy, informed, and educated and feel taken care of all in a single day's work.

On this day, though, I was just tired. The voice inside my head was yawning, and I didn't want to talk to so many people. An upbeat medical student was with me and we went to the postpartum rooms to examine a baby together. Sometimes you walk into a postpartum room and the family is half asleep with all the lights off, the TV blaring, and the baby dressed in an outfit consisting of more than a dozen snaps. This can present several barriers to performing a full physical exam because you need a well-lit room and a naked baby to make sure the exam is complete. In this moment, though, the parents were awake, the lights were on, and the baby was already unwrapped in the crib. I let a yawn slip out. At least the baby was undressed and it was bright—I could do this. The conditions were perfect to approach this baby, examine them in a matter of minutes, and escape back to the hallway for a micro nap against the wall while I droned on about the typical findings to my energetic trainee.

I smiled at the family, asked if this was a good time to see the baby, and went about the standard maneuvers I've performed time and time again for the infant exam. Listening to the heart and lungs, then going from head to toe checking all the body parts. The medical student was watching me eagerly, as was the family as I took in their new baby. Often, I try not to announce gender when I enter an infant's room, instead calling the infant "baby" until the family invites me to say boy or girl. The last place I look is in the diaper, and most of the time a parent's preferred gender identity for their baby matches the baby's sex organs. I undid this baby's diaper and began assessing the penis and scrotum. I felt for the testicles because I wanted to make sure both were in the scrotal sac. It was my routine testicular exam—but it was not routine for the family or my medical student. The birth parent, half joking and half serious, asked me point-blank, "Why are you touching my baby's 'balls'?" The medical student burst into nervous laughter as I palpated the scrotal sac. At that moment I realized my inner voice had fallen asleep so I was silently touching a baby's privates; this family deserved an explanation, and my medical student needed to see how I would explain this.

It was important to explain why I touch all babies' testicles (I'll go into that more in a minute). Now I strive to explain my initial physical exam findings in detail, and so I spend my days in the nursery, physically examining babies and verbally explaining that to my medical students, and I hope they learn a lot, and I hope you will too as I give you the infant physical exam. Checking in on your baby's parts and your pediatrician's smarts.

The baby is just born. Wow. You've been thinking about parenting, wondering about delivery, and now here is a baby. Many times, the baby is placed on a birth parent's chest. Wriggling and crying, and geez they look a little weirder than expected. Aren't babies supposed to be cute and round. Why is the head so cone shaped? What's all this white stuff? Where did all this blood come from? As I like to say, the exchange of bodily fluids is about to get real.

The time after delivery is generally not restful in the hospital. Childbirth is both a miracle and a major medical event. It's important to monitor the health of both the mother and the baby. Lots of recovery is mixed with lots of learning about this new human, their anatomy, and the basic functioning of their body. Ultrasounds and blood testing of the pregnant parent can tell us a lot about the health of the growing infant. Until we meet your baby, we don't know the specifics of how their ears are placed, what their butt crack looks like, or if they might have an extra pinky finger sticking out of their hand. The time right after delivery is a time of transition—to creating a new family structure, to building a relationship with a nonverbal human, and to learning that parenting a newborn requires vigilance and decision-making from the moment your tiny human is born.

There is a medical definition of the term *transition* when it refers to a newborn. Transition is defined as a very complex adaptation from being supported by the placenta in a fluid-filled environment to coming out and breathing air with a fresh set of lungs. That new set of lungs must now provide oxygen to the baby's body, and their brand spanking new heart must start its lifelong job of pumping blood to the body. If this transition is delayed, a baby generally needs help immediately to jumpstart this intricate heart and lung dance. So, even if being in the hospital is not the best for relationship building and rest, it is a time to ensure the baby gets examined and receives the newborn screenings they need for a healthy start. A healthy start is what you want for a lasting relationship.

In this chapter, we will discuss the newborn exam (you will hear my inner monologue on this) and what happens to a birth parent's body. The next chapter (Chapter 5) will be about newborn screens: vitamin K, erythromycin, the critical congenital heart defect screen (the name says it all!), state newborn screens, hearing screens, monitoring for jaundice, and the hepatitis B vaccine. This is a lot to get done for a baby who likely will be in the hospital for a total of 24 to 72 hours. However, these evaluations are essential for making sure you have the time to bond with your healthy baby when you are discharged.

A Baby's Body

I've started moving away from using the word *normal* to describe an infant's exam. If a baby has an ear pit—a tiny dimple by their ear—I'll note it as a finding. And while most infants don't have ear pits, it's not like it's abnormal to find one. It's just a range of what's *typical* (my substitute for normal) in an infant exam. Your baby has a red blotchy rash with areas of raised white bumps? We call that erythema toxicum, a scary name for a benign baby rash that pops up and moves around the body wherever it can find hair follicles. Found on most babies? Yes. Normal? Sure, but it's not abnormal when you don't have it. So, again, I like to say erythema toxicum is the most typical newborn rash. Because many newborns develop strange-looking skin rashes, it's also typical to need to use photo editing software when taking pictures of them.

As mentioned earlier, I also make a point of talking through my examination of a baby. I have been guilty of trying to act like a ninja and maneuver myself stealthily around the birth parent and the baby. Slipping my hands into the bassinet for an exam and then silently making my way out of the room to let the family sleep. But, having been questioned for touching a baby's "balls," I now want you to know why I'm going to be touching your infant's genitalia. Sometimes I find my mostly monotone talking and explanations help lull tired families to sleep, and I'm happy to be the white noise they need in recovery. What's most important is that they understand their baby's body.

My exams always start with watching the newborn before I put my hands on them. Babies love to be all scrunched up. When I unwrap them from a swaddle, most will still have their arms and legs flexed in a "I'm still stuck in the womb" sort of positioning. Then they generally kick out their limbs in all directions, exploring the freedom of some extra space. These movements aren't coordinated. They happen in fits and starts with tiny jerks evident in their wiggling limbs. Humans are born without their brains fully developed. We are going to talk later about how millions upon millions of connections need to form in the first few months to year after birth as their brains develop. I receive a lot of questions from families about those jerky movements or the baby being "jittery" when I see them for the first time. I want you to know that I expect most babies to have jerky movements early on. This is because the myelin—or covering outside of the nerve cells—that helps them communicate seamlessly with each other (nerve cells love to talk) isn't developed in babies. When you watch a baby start to gain control of their muscles, it begins from the center out and from the top down. This control is attained from the nerve cells being myelinated and talking more easily with each other. It's a beautiful thing to watch if you have the pleasure of living with an infant. How they gain head control, then trunk control as they roll and sit, finally holding their head up; then, it's out to the limbs to drag or crawl and finally down to the fingers as they attain fine motor control. That nerve control is what we celebrate as infants reach their developmental milestones. The beautiful blossoming of their brains.

The Heart of the Matter

I don't start by touching the baby's head. I've noticed most babies will cry when I examine their heads. It makes me feel like they all must have a massive headache after delivery. Of course I can't ask them, and we wouldn't treat it with anything but skin-to-skin with their families and feedings. So I always begin by placing my stethoscope on them to listen to their heart and lungs. I start with the heart. I want to hear that cartoon "lub dub" sound. What you might not know is the heart has 4 main chambers and acts as a big pump to get blood to the lungs and the body. The heartbeat isn't the sound of the heart muscle itself contracting, because the heart is one big, special, constantly active muscle. The beating sound is the blood flow and the plumbing of the heart. The heart contains valves that open and close to make sure blood keeps flowing from the lungs to the body. You want blood to go from the right side of the heart into the lungs and return to the left side of the heart and get pumped to the body. Just like there are 4 chambers of the heart, there are 4 main valves that keep the blood flow steady.

The Heart

Here's a drawing of a heart pumping away and taking over the job of the placenta to make sure the body gets the oxygen-rich blood it needs.

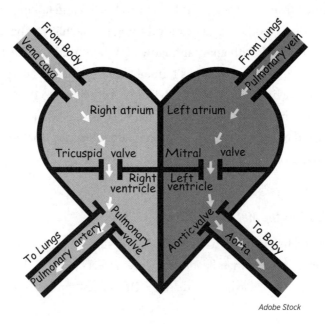

Adobe Stock

So there are 2 things I want to hear a heart do: beat regularly without missing a beat. Again, I want lub dub, lub dub, not lub dub … silence … lub dub. I expect the baby to have a very fast heartbeat, which reacts and gets faster if they are touched or crying, and it slows down in sleep. But I want to make sure they have steady beats, at a regular rate. If they do not, I'll order an electrocardiogram (ECG or EKG). This test will help me see the baby's heartbeat on paper and watch the magical electricity that coordinates all of its muscular contractions.

The second thing I want to listen for is something called a murmur. That's not like a whisper you hear when playing the telephone game. It's a sound that occurs when blood flow is turbulent or unsteady; this can be typical or a sign the blood is not flowing the way it's supposed to. The 4 chambers of the heart should have no connections between them, and the valves should be water-tight, really blood-tight and not allow for blood to go anywhere but the lungs first, body second. I don't want to listen to a heart and hear lub-shubbb-dub or hear this rumbling shhhhhh behind a lub dub. I just want a lub dub. No static please.

That said, even if I hear a shubbbb or a shhhh (aka a murmur), that's not always a bad thing. When a baby is inside the womb, they actually don't need to send a lot of blood to the lungs because the placenta does all the heavy lifting in supplying oxygen and nutrients to the body. The placenta acts as the lungs for the fetus. As such, the growing baby sends blood away from the heart and lungs to feed other parts of the body. There are special fetal connections that help blood bypass the lungs and go to the body and the placenta. In medicine, we can't call these connections simple things like connection 1 or 2. We have fancier names such as a patent ductus arteriosus (PDA) and a patent foramen ovale (PFO). So we name it, then abbreviate it to make it as confusing as possible for those not trained in the language of medicine. Parlez-vous neonatal anatomy anyone? You don't have to know all the names of the different connections of heart vessels. If a doctor hears a murmur in a newborn, it's usually their body adjusting to having to circulate oxygenated blood on their own. This is not something you want a baby to be doing after birth, so these connections will usually close after the baby is born. When this happens, the heart needs to work harder, as it is now responsible for getting blood to the lungs and to the whole body as well. This is how incredible it is when a baby takes their first breath—the lungs fill with air, the blood vessels in the lungs open up, the right side of the heart sends them blood, and a whole new circulation is established. All within minutes.

The heart is the steady drum of circulation. It works closely with the lungs to make sure the body gets the blood it needs. If there is a murmur, your pediatrician or pediatric professional should let you know if they think it needs more investigation. If so, an ultrasound of the heart called an echocardiogram may be ordered.

Take a Deep Breath In

Once I'm finished with the heart, I listen to the lungs. Essentially, I want to hear nothing or the lungs to be "clear." We say that a lot: "The lungs sound clear." But clear of what? Since the lungs don't really have a job in the womb (thanks again, magical and mystical placenta), they are filled with fluid. It's important to know that that fluid is not the amniotic fluid the baby swims around in. It's a special lung fluid that helps the lungs grow and expand—the lung makes it all on its own. At the time of delivery, *something* during labor—we aren't exactly sure what, but we have some ideas about fluctuating hormones playing a role—tells the baby's body to start absorbing that fluid so the lungs can fill with air. If a baby's lungs don't sound clear we likely think of them as having some of that fluid remaining—this is called transient (short time period) tachypnea (fast breathing) of the newborn. We like to abbreviate this as TTN (we love acronyms!).

This is the most common reason a baby might need support after delivery. It can't really be diagnosed on examination, but a chest X-ray shows the fluid. Listen, if your baby ever needs an X-ray, ask the doctor to walk you through what they are seeing and why the X-ray is important. For TTN, you can see fluid in a common area between the lobes of the lung; that and a patchy haziness around the heart usually makes TTN the diagnosis. With a little support or just watchful waiting, the lungs will become clear.

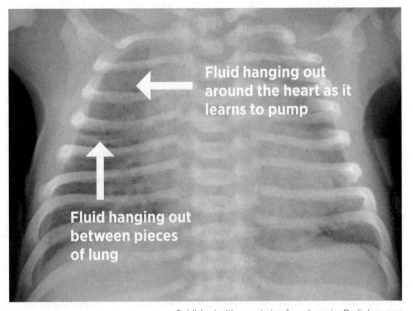

Fluid hanging out around the heart as it learns to pump

Fluid hanging out between pieces of lung

Published with permission from LearningRadiology.com

As a neonatologist, I could talk about lung sounds all day, as there are other conditions in babies related to the lungs having to adapt to circulating blood and getting air filled. But many of the lung issues I see aren't typical for a healthy newborn, so I'll spare you the medicalese on those conditions. I just want the lungs to be clear.

But breathing isn't just about the lungs, it's also about the airway. I will often touch my neck and feel the cartilage there, demonstrating to parents the piece of my airway I can touch. I'll also refer to it as the windpipe. I took a minute to touch it now as I was writing and it's a hard cartilage with some bumpiness forming a tube for me to breath in and out of. We like to call it the trachea. As I'm placing a stethoscope on the lungs to make sure they are clear, I'm also watching the baby breath to make sure the airway is open and air can enter and exit the body smoothly. I want it to look easy.

Often, newborns use their bellies to breath, and so I'll see the belly going in and out as they take breaths. This is due, to a certain extent, to the movement of the belly muscles, but it is related more to a very large muscle called the diaphragm that separates the lungs from the intestines. You also have lesser known and much smaller muscles between your ribs called the intercostals. Sounds like a fun vacation spot; every day when I examine a baby I'm visiting the intercostals and checking in. Much like when you are on vacation, those muscles should be relaxed, so I shouldn't see them pulling in between the ribs. That could be a sign the baby is using too much energy to breath and won't have it for other things like eating and bonding. I also don't want to see them using muscles around their windpipe and doing something called tracheal tugging. Sometimes, I don't even need to put my stethoscope on a baby to know if they have a problem with their airway. Babies make a sort of gasping sound when it's difficult for them to bring air into their bodies. It sounds like a seal bark, whereas most newborn cries make them sound like sheep. You want a sheep-sounding baby and not a seal-sounding one. Yes, we have a name for this—stridor—and it tells us something might be blocking the airway. Sometimes, when those hard cartilage rings are not fully formed, the airway can collapse on itself. Or there can be some tissue or something else blocking the airway. Generally, when we hear those sounds but the baby looks well and can get good oxygen into their body, we don't worry too much. We might ask subspecialists called ear, nose, and throat (ENT) doctors to come and listen too. The most common reasons for stridor are having areas of weak cartilage in the airway that collapse when the baby breaths in, making that high-pitched huuuuup or seal-like gasping sound. Because the baby's airway is small, they usually outgrow this over time, but having the ENT doctor check them and sometimes even put a camera in their nose to see their airway is helpful.

The sound I probably get asked about the most is a baby's snoring. I can tell you right after delivery, a lot of babies sound snorty or snotty. Babies like to breathe out of their noses. If they have anything in their nose such as vernix (the cheesy lotion they are born with), blood, or [insert body fluid here], they will likely sound like they are snoring. That snorting sound can also occur when they are awake and active. Also, newborns generally have a lot of pressure on their heads and faces during delivery, so they are a little more swollen at first. Should you suction their nose? If they are otherwise comfortable and pink, you don't need to. Sometimes sticking something up the nose only causes it to have more inflammation or swelling, which prolongs their nasal congestion. If you see boogers or blood, sure, get it out with that classic blue bulb syringe you will be given. But if you don't see anything and they aren't using extra muscles to breath, I generally let whatever it is work itself out. Sometimes you can spray some sterile saline up the nose. In theory, salt-rich water is meant to break apart any mucus that might be stuck up there. In practice, it's probably more of a rinse, but it might be effective to do something.

Lastly, I can say with certainty your baby does not have allergies. I get asked about babies being allergic to things like dust or pollen. To have allergies, you need to have a robust immune system that has identified things in the environment and decided it doesn't like them. Babies do not have really sophisticated immune responses because their immune system is not well developed. So a baby having a runny nose because of an allergy—that's not really a thing.

Putting Our Heads Together

Even though a newborn doesn't like it when I touch their heads, I do it. Because the brain is arguably the most important organ and I want to check in on it. Also, did you know your skull is not just 1 bone? In fact, it's 22 bones making up the face and encasing the brain. The skull is a very important bone for protection, but babies need a little wiggle room. Out of these 22 bones, there are 5 bones that I actually feel in the infant's head: the frontal, parietal, and occipital bones. The frontal bone is—you got it—in the front of the head. It largely makes up the forehead. The parietal bones are large bones that make up the sides and top of the head and come together in the middle of the skull. The occipital bone takes up the rear and sometimes makes a real point of it, meaning it's typical for the bone to end in a little shelf (called the bathrocephaly—we really have a lot of names for the noggin).

These 4 large bones have joints in between them. Because these joints don't move like your elbow or your knee, we insist on confusing laypeople by calling them sutures. Little areas of the bone that are stitched together by some cartilage, creating the soft spots of the head. The anterior fontanelle, or the very large soft spot right at the top of the head toward the forehead, is the joint where the frontal and parietal bones meet. Soft spots disappear over time because as the brain grows, the bones grow, and eventually the skull becomes hard to protect the brain. Again, we'll go over this in later chapters, but the brain is growing *rapidly*, maybe the fastest it will ever grow in your human's life. Three-fourths of brain growth occurs in the first 2 years after birth.

The reason why the bones of the head aren't fused is they are meant to take a beating coming out into the world. They can bend and smush together and not break. This leads most newborn babies' heads to have what we call *molding*. Think of shaping clay into a cone shape to fit through the cervix and vagina. That's sort of what a newborn's head looks like; the term *cone head* also gets passed around a fair amount. That doesn't mean your baby's *head* is malleable like clay. You can't physically push it back into a nice round shape. Time and gravity can do that and we don't recommend applying more pressure to an infant's head, as they have already been through it. Just as the head changed shape to enter the world, it will change back ... almost all of the time.

Except when it doesn't. Because sometimes it won't. While I'm seemingly massaging a baby's head as they cry after birth, I'm also feeling each bone and the sutures or joints between them. I want to make sure the joints are open to allow for growth of the brain; if they aren't, I want to look more closely for something called craniosynostosis. Cranio stands for the cranium or the brain, syn for fused, os refers to bones, and tosis means some sort of condition, usually not a good one (for example, halitosis means bad breath, yuck, but new word! As an aside, my favorite word is mondegreen, which refers to mishearing music lyrics. It has nothing to do with a baby's head, just wanted to share). In craniosynostosis, the joints are fused in the skull, which does not allow for the brain or the head to grow properly. If the head is misshapen because of craniosynostosis, time isn't going to allow it to grow well. So, early diagnosis and tracking of brain growth is very important for these babies. Additionally, sometimes when one of the sutures or joints closes early, it means there is something genetic going on and the closure is part of a larger syndrome or condition. If I feel a joint that seems fused in the skull, I like to let my genetics colleagues know to give your baby the best start possible. Sometimes though these changes in the skull are just random. The most common joint that closes early extends from the soft spot across the top of the head to the back of the skull and is called the sagittal suture. So during typical exams of healthy babies, I'm always feeling a little extra for that opening.

I'll bet you didn't realize just how much goes into touching your baby's head. In fact, I'm not even done writing about the head.

Where Are You Headed With This?

I will admit that even if the baby doesn't have something rarer like craniosynostosis, sometimes the head shape doesn't become a perfectly round circle as they grow. But the shape generally is far better by the end of the first week. If you don't believe me, look at pictures of your older kids or your relatives' or friends' newborns on day 1 (sans hat; hats, especially those with sparkle, always make the baby's head look adorable) and then look again on day 7. The difference is dramatic. The face starts out a little puffy at birth because of being beaten up, and that, coupled with the cone-shaped head, makes babies look weird. Plus, keep in mind that the head is really squeezed and pushed on during delivery, so often that leads to bruising on the head. Yes, bruising. It's so common it's one of those things we love to test medical students on: exactly what types of bruising or hematomas a baby has on their scalp. If a student doctor or medical student is caring for your baby that day, you can test their knowledge by asking them if your baby has a cephalohematoma or caput. These names are designations for where on the scalp or around the skull bones the bleeding or bruising occurs. The cephalohematoma is restricted to a bone and so you feel a little lump over 1 of the 4 major skull bones. The caput is like a cap. It can extend over bones and is lumplike and a little firm. Bigger bleeds can also occur and these are called subgaleal bleeds. These are very serious and very boggy, and they generally extend down the neck. If you tap them, you can see the blood underneath, and babies with these may need admission to a neonatal intensive care unit for monitoring of the bleeding. Luckily, they are more rare, and cephalohematomas and caputs are the most common bumps on the baby's head. These also should be essentially gone by 1 week of age.

However, it's not like a week after delivery parents stop stressing about their baby's head shape. It's just that the reasons for concern change. Remember, the skull bones aren't fused into place and can still move around. One of the most common misshapen head conditions we see is called plagiocephaly, which means the back of the head is flat on one side. It's reported that up to half of parents notice some head flattening on their baby. While this can be a byproduct of the delivery, it often appears around 2 to 3 months of age and can take 2 to 3 years to resolve itself. Digging back into your knowledge of geometry (if you are an architect or a mathematician or a similar smartie, know that I'm not and teaching my kids the difference between a triangle and square is about as far as I've dived into the study of shapes), babies with plagiocephaly often have a parallelogram-shaped head. One part of the forehead is shoved forward while the back of the head on the other side sticks out.

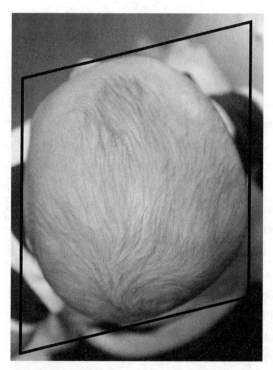

Used with permission from Dias MS, Samson T, Rizk EB, Governale LS, Richtsmeier JT; American Academy of Pediatrics Section on Neurologic Surgery and Section on Plastic and Reconstructive Surgery. Identifying the misshapen head: craniosynostosis and related disorders. *Pediatrics*. 2020;146(3):e2020015511.

Prenatally, if the baby was bigger, had to share the womb with another baby (twinning), or was jammed in the pelvis in a certain way, they might have this head shape no matter what you do. But there are things you can do to try to prevent a flat head if it hasn't already happened. Frequent positional changes help, so moving the baby around in your arms with different holds is a nice way to switch up the pressure on the loosey goosey skull bones. Early tummy time—after a baby is a few weeks old—is a good way to take pressure off the head. Sometimes, it's not even an issue with the head really, but the muscles of the baby's neck are tight and pulling the head to one side. This is called torticollis, which sometimes can be felt as a knot in the neck on examination.

If you've been obsessively trying to prevent a flat head, the first thing to do is stop stressing over the perfect head shape. Remember, around half of babies will have some flattening, and as long as their brain is growing and their development is typical, your worry-o-meter should be low. If you are already making sure to position the baby in different ways, you are doing a ton of work to help prevent this. If you notice an issue with the neck, asking your pediatrician for neck exercises or having a physical therapy consult to get your baby's neck stretched out might be the key to remodeling their head shape. If those things don't work, there are baby helmets. Baby helmets aren't like bike helmets; they are braces made to push the skull bones back to a rounded shape. The evidence for this is questionable, because it's unclear if using a helmet really helps reshape the head, or if time is what babies really need for the head to take shape. Have a serious discussion with a trusted doctor and an unfulfilling and painful discussion with your insurance company before investing in one of these. The helmet must be custom fitted, and for it to "work," the baby needs to wear it up to 23 hours a day. So it's an investment in money, time, and comfort for your growing little one. The good news here is surgery is rarely, if ever, needed to help reshape the future of your baby's head.

It's a Reflex

My favorite exam move is called the Galant. It's when you rub your finger on the side of the back of a baby and they wiggle their butt toward your hand. It looks like they are dancing, and it is lovely. Babies have a lot of these reflexes or involuntary movements. Recognizing them on exam tells you a lot about how their nervous system is programmed and will give you clues to their development as they grow.

Probably the most popular reflex is the startle or Moro reflex. This occurs when the baby is spooked and suddenly throws their arms out to the side and then into the center. Imagine that they are getting ready to give a big awkward hug, or have just jumped from a plane and are getting their parachute in place. What's important to me is that they have this reflex, and that both sides of the body seem to move in unison. Another adorable reflex is the palmar grasp. This is where the baby will hold anything you put in their hands. Parents love to sneak a finger in there and talk about how their baby wants to hold their hand, inviting them to be loved and recognized. I'm all about the palmar grasp as a love language, and I want to see it on exam. Similarly, placing anything within reach of the toes will elicit the plantar grasp and the baby will grab it. (This motion is also helpful when parents need to clean their baby's toys at the end of the day and don't want to bend down.)

Other common reflexes I look for include the stepping reflex, where the baby will literally march on any surface you place them. Rooting occurs when a baby tries to suck anything placed against their cheek or lips. It can look like they are trying to eat their fingers or the swaddle blanket they are wrapped in and is actually a good sign that the baby *is* hungry! Lastly, the tonic neck reflex, or more aptly named fencer reflex, occurs when you turn the baby's head, and the arm on the side they are looking toward stretches out while the opposite arm flexes inward. It's like they are extending a sword in self-defense. On guard! This reflex doesn't tell you if they will be good at fencing when they grow up, but you can decide if you want them to try it when they are older. All of these reflexes, as fun and cute as they are, usually go away by the end of the first year after birth. Your pediatrician will help track them for you.

COMMON INFANT REFLEXES AND WHEN THEY DISAPPEAR

REFLEX	AGE WHEN REFLEX APPEARS	AGE WHEN REFLEX DISAPPEARS
Stepping	Birth	2 months
Rooting	Birth	4 months
Palmar grasp	Birth	5–6 months
Moro reflex	Birth	2 months
Tonic neck reflex	Birth	5–7 months
Plantar grasp	Birth	9–12 months

Adapted from *Caring for Your Baby and Young Child: Birth to Age 5,* 7th Edition (Copyright © 2019 American Academy of Pediatrics).

While reflexes tell you a lot about a baby's brain, there is one more exam move I like to do to test their muscle tone. It often freaks out families, so I'll tell you about it before you see me do it. I love to pick up babies and usually sit them up first (gives me a good view of the noggin), but then I put my hand over their chest and belly and hold

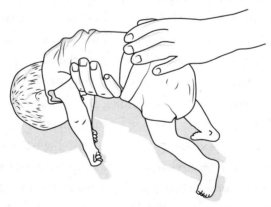

Exam maneuver most likely to freak out families. In this illustration the baby has poor muscle tone (hypotonia). Note the C-shape with inability to lift the head or butt.

Used with permission from Huff HV, Huff KR. Hypotonia. In: American Academy of Pediatrics. *Berkowitz's Pediatrics: A Primary Care Approach.* Berkowitz CD, ed. 6th ed. American Academy of Pediatrics; 2020:961.

them up with one hand. Babies are not fragile; this will not break them. In fact, this tells me so much about their strength and muscle tone, I usually don't skip it. I like to see that they can hold their back up in a straight line and don't just fall into a C-shape over my palm.

Let's Face It

From head to face. I'm looking to see how the eyes and ears are positioned. I check the ears to look for skin tags or pits, which are commonly seen. I'll then check the nose, making sure the baby is breathing from it and it's not too crushed from delivery. If I see boogers, I'll show families how to suction them out. I only use a bulb suction or one of those nasal aspirators if I see something in the nose. Otherwise, over-suctioning a baby's tiny nose can cause inflammation and snorting you don't want.

I should be able to open the mouth easily. There shouldn't be teeth, but if there are, I'm not that impressed. Natal or neonatal teeth are more typical than you think. They are generally baby teeth, and adult teeth will still come in when it's time. I don't stress about them unless they are affecting feeding or are loose. I will then consult a dentist and request that families prepare for the tooth fairy to come early. We want babies to eat well, and loose teeth can be swallowed and choked on so aren't safe to leave in. Remember, when you summon the tooth fairy, there shouldn't be any pillows in the crib or sleep area, so you will need to be more creative about how to celebrate the baby's first lost tooth. While I'm in the mouth examining, I'll also massage the gums, feeling for the presence of a cyst, which can be on the gum line. I'll then run my finger over the roof of the mouth checking to see that the palate is intact. Having a cleft palate—or hole in the room of the mouth—can also affect feeding, so it's important to diagnose. The lip can also have a cleft, but that's easier to see by looking at the baby. To feel the inside of the mouth, I offer a gloved finger for the baby to suck on. Usually, I can get the baby to do a nice rhythmic suck, but if I can't, I acknowledge that a gloved finger doesn't look, feel, or taste like a birth parent or a bottle of milk and so I don't hold a disorganized suck against a new baby. Also, while the suck is a reflex, some newborns are still working out how they can suck, swallow, and breath all at once. Preterm infants in particular need extra support to sort themselves out, so often I recommend that parents of early term (37 weeks) and preterm infants stay for feeding support for as long as they can before discharge.

Necking

Babies often have no visible neck. Their heads are held on by who knows what. Plus, we know the neck can't really support babies' big heads. There will be more on that in the sleep chapter, but that's why you have to support their head when you hold them. I always move a baby's puffy adorable cheeks and double chins out of the way to really see the neck. I'll look at the neck muscles. Sometimes you can see or feel enlarged muscles making the baby at risk for torticollis. I like to look at the back of the neck as well because it's common to have a nevus simplex there. A nevus essentially refers to a birthmark, and simplex is simple, usually just a flat pink patch. Nevus simplex has a lot of names, including salmon patch, or if it is on the back of the neck, a stork bite. I love to tell a birth parent that the stork has delivered this beautiful baby into the world. Having tried this joke on many families, very few ever think it's funny right after delivering a baby.

Chest and Belly

Generally, at this point I've already listened to the chest, taking in the sounds of the heart and the motion of the chest wall as a baby breathes. I'll also look at the nipples—are there 2? More than 2? Having extra nipples is not uncommon and generally they occur on what's called the milk line. Think of a cat nursing their baby kittens; given they have multiple kittens in their litter, they need more than

2 breasts with nipples to feed them. It's believed the extra nipples are just a vestige of being evolved mammals. It's hard to tell the difference between an accessory or extra nipple and a congenital nevus or mole right at delivery, so often I'll note the mark but won't make the call that it's a nipple. I'll let time and puberty (aka hormonal changes later on) decide. Also, breast buds are pretty common irrespective of gender assigned at birth. The same hormones that helped mom deliver also influence the baby. For these swollen lumps, resist the urge to press on them. You want to just let them shrink on their own. Any redness or swelling of the breast tissue needs evaluation, but a tiny leakage of milk in the first few weeks can be normal. Let your pediatrician help monitor if they make you nervous.

Moving on to the belly. It should be soft and the only organ in it that someone should be able to feel is the liver. The liver is a hard, regenerative organ under the right ribs; your stomach is on the left. The edge of the liver can sometimes be felt popping out under the lung. The spleen, kidneys, and intestines should not be as easy to feel. The belly button is also of concern to us. Not whether there is one, because the umbilical cord is still hanging out where it was after delivery. We cannot determine if your baby will have an innie or an outie and there isn't really a way to control for this. Remember, it is a cosmetic thing. What I *can* tell you is if there is a small hernia or break in the muscle wall close to the umbilical cord. A baby will never be born with a 6-pack because the abdominal muscles aren't strong or well formed. Many babies have something called diastasis recti. This is a typical condition for newborns where the abdominal walls looks separated, so when the baby strains or cries, a little bit of the belly pokes through in the middle and looks like a sausage. As the baby gets bigger and starts to try to sit up and move that muscle, the diastasis recti should close or be much less visible. This is not the same as diastasis recti caused by pregnancy and requiring physical therapy and maybe a tummy tuck. More on that when we talk about the birth parent's physical exam after delivery.

Feeling Hip

One thing you should witness all pediatricians do is a hip exam. The hip is a large joint, and when you are older one that really helps you get around and bears a lot of weight. As a baby, they won't be putting a lot of pressure on their hips, but the doctor will when they examine them. Why? Because the hip is a ball and socket joint. The ball is the head of a femur or the leg bone, and the socket is the rounded cavity of the pelvic bone. Sometimes the femur can get free from the pelvis, the ball doesn't land in the hole it's supposed to, and the joint is not intact. Since a baby doesn't walk, it's not going to notice this. And hormones make it so the joints of both the birth parent and the baby are pretty loose, so with some extra flexibility and no weight bearing this hip dislocation (aka hip joint not being in the right spot) causes no pain for the infant. It will however be a pain if the femur doesn't get relocated back into the right spot. It can cause walking issues later in life. Pediatricians check for hip joint stability by doing maneuvers to see if the hip is dislocated and to attempt to move it back into the joint if they find it is out. If a pediatrician feels like the hip joint is dislocated, we will call our friends in orthopedic surgery to help us monitor and brace the joint. Putting on a specific type of brace called a Pavlik harness is the most common way to address this relatively common issue.

Risk factors for hip dislocation include something called the 4 Fs.

1. **F**irstborn babies

2. **F**emales (Girls are at higher risk.)

3. **F**eet-first (Meaning that the baby was breech or head up sometime in the third trimester. This will automatically get you a hip ultrasound when the baby is around 6 weeks old. Something to know about breech babes.)

4. **F**amily history (Someone else in the family had hip dysplasia, meaning the hip joint wasn't together as a baby.)

So let you doctors feel hip…like literally watch as they feel the hips and let you know about the joint.

The Private Parts

I call this section of the book "the private parts." I want to be clear, though, when I am talking about your baby's private parts I use the anatomical names in my exam. Because penis, scrotum, testicles, vulva, clitoris, and vagina are not dirty words. They are not bad jokes or off-limit topics to discuss in a physical. They are a part of our bodies, and when examining a baby I want to make sure these parts—at least outwardly—are healthy.

For babies born with a vulva and vagina, I'll begin just by looking at the vulva. Next, I'll pull apart the labia majora—the large skin folds—to look at the clitoris and vagina beneath. I'll make sure the clitoris is an appropriate size and the urethra appears to be coming out of it. I'll also inspect the vagina. Is there a bulge coming out of it? Anything sticking out of the vagina requires further investigation. I've seen bluish bulges representing a stretched hymen or a prolapsed uterus. If I'm worried about something like that, a pelvic ultrasound is the first step in my workup. That said, if there is a fleshy looking skin tag with a slight bulge from the vagina or near the labia minora—the smaller skin folds in the labia majora—this can be a normal hormonal response to delivery. These are important to note because they can freak out families if they are big, but they tend to shrink over time and not be as visible. There isn't anything further to assess and I can reassure parents that these findings are typical. What's also typical is vaginal discharge after delivery. Sometimes there is some blood, resembling a sort of light period. Other times, there is a thick white vaginal discharge. For the first few weeks, this is typical, again (you guessed it) resulting from changing hormones after delivery.

For babies born with a penis, I look at the size and also at where the urethra (or pee hole) comes out. I expect it to be at the tip of the penis, but if it is anywhere on the shaft of the penis, the infant may have something called hypospadias. Male infants are born with a foreskin, and I don't try to pull the foreskin back to get a look at the entire head of the penis, because the foreskin tends to be more adherent in the first few months after birth and pulling it back can cause trauma. After assessing the penis, I look at the scrotum. I'm looking at the size and shape of the scrotal sac. I want to see if it appears symmetric, indicating there are 2 testicles within it. The testicle is an organ that takes a journey to wind up in the scrotum. Ovaries and testicles have similar origins and, based on hormonal cues, these sex organs end up in different places. Ovaries are told to stay put, and testicles are asked to go on a venture south. As with any journey, it has some obstacles.

For the first 8 weeks of its existence, the primordial testicle hangs out by the kidney. The kidneys are a super cool organ, and I imagine the testicle is sad to leave them. But given they need a cooler environment as they mature, the scrotum offers more time to hang outside of the body at a lower temperature. So, they make their way outside the warm belly. After the first 2 months of fetal development, hormones tell the testicle to begin to go to something called the inguinal region. This is the area where the upper thigh meets the belly. The testicle has to slip down through the inguinal canal to make its way into the scrotum. This canal should close by the time of a term birth. Again, lots of hormones and different tissues and processes are involved. The testicle can stall and sometimes gets stuck in the belly, or it gets stuck in the inguinal canal—so close to the scrotum but not quite there. The inguinal canal itself sometimes cannot close properly, so some of the intestines or bowel could slip into the scrotum as well. This is called an inguinal hernia. Hernias in the private area are much more common in babies with a penis, scrotum, and testicles, but they can develop in those with a vulva as well if the inguinal canal doesn't close. For all babies, a hernia is usually an asymmetric bulge on one side of the body. Again, symmetry is important to note and look for on physical exam.

When a testicle is not down at birth, the medical staff at the birth hospital will counsel your pediatrician to watch for it to fall. If both testicles are held up, an ultrasound is required right after birth to make sure the testicles are present and accounted for. If, by about age 5 to 6 months, a testicle hasn't come down on its own, the testicle is unlikely to complete the journey and surgical assistance is required. Similarly, hernias also require surgery to close the inguinal canal and keep the intestine in the belly. The thought of any surgery in a baby is scary, which is why I always stress the importance of having surgeries performed at children's hospitals trained to deal with these types of relatively common procedures. These simpler repairs are usually outpatient procedures, and the baby can recover at home.

I Surmise I Should Circumcise?

Do you want to circumcise your baby? If you ask me whether you should, I'll immediately counter with a question: Do you want to? Because circumcision is not required of you.

My husband and I had big debates about piercing our daughter's ears. I had my ears pierced as an infant, and I wanted hers to be pierced as well. My husband thought this was not something you put a baby through, and she could get her ears pierced when she was older and could decide if that's what she wanted. I'm still frustrated I didn't have them pierced as an infant, because now as a school-aged kid, it feels like the wrong time to put her through something painful. There is a key difference though between putting a hole in your baby's earlobe and taking off their foreskin. This is coming from someone who has 5 empty holes in her ears and only 2 filled with earrings. Yes, the penis is a more private and sensitive part of the body than the ear, but removing a foreskin is not something you can do at your local mall. And when the head of the penis heals, new skin doesn't grow back. However, just like getting a baby's ears pierced, getting it done early means the recovery will be quicker, and likely the pain from the event won't be remembered. There is a more time-sensitive nature to the circumcision decision. If not done right after delivery, more and different types of anesthesia will be needed to ensure the procedure is comfortable.

There are also some slight benefits to being circumcised. Circumcision can reduce the chance of already rare penile cancer, but it can also reduce the chance of developing infections in that area—whether it be urinary tract infections or infections of the foreskin that can travel down the shaft of the penis. No one likes to think their infant may have a sex life in the future (but let's hope they do), and circumcision can also help decrease the transmission of sexually transmitted infections. But these advantages aren't so compelling that everyone should undergo circumcision—again, it's a personal choice. The American Academy of Pediatrics gets a lot of flak at their national meetings for saying there are benefits to circumcision and every family should have the ability to get the procedure if they think it's right for their infant with a penis. This is not a ringing endorsement—it's a way of saying you have the right to choose—and an acknowledgment of the science behind circumcision. It is true that if you decide to have your infant circumcised, they don't get a voice or a choice. This is true of many decisions made in parenting an infant. Talk with your family about circumcision, think of your own values, and make a choice that is in line with your personal desires. This is an area where you can ignore the noise and focus on your family's wishes.

A Birth Parent's Body After Delivery

Birth parents tend not to undergo an extensive physical like the baby right after delivery. If the delivery was vaginal, the vagina gets inspected, stitches are generally in place, and your belly gets pushed on a few times before you go. If the delivery was a cesarean section

(c-section), the incision is checked and again your belly gets pushed
on a bit, but then you are discharged. There is a disparity in the care
of the birth parent and baby after leaving the hospital. While the baby
will get around 9 visits in the first year after birth, the birth parent
generally has a 4- to 6-week postpartum visit, and unless they schedule
something after that with their obstetrician/gynecologist, that might
be it. It's important to know there are changes to a birth parent's body,
changes evident on physical exams that are typical after having a baby.
But typical does not mean it's all ok. Peeing on yourself every time you
laugh? That can be typical after having a baby, but it doesn't have to be
accepted or considered the norm. There are things you can do to help
your body heal from one of the most intense physical exercises it has
ever done. Let's talk about some fourth trimester body changes and
think about whether you need to undergo a physical to address them.

The Brain

While we spend a lot of time feeling your newborn's head, there
needs to be a focus on what's going on inside a birth parent's head.
Postpartum mood disorders are common and will be covered in
greater depth when we talk about feeding a baby. Aside from the
hormonal and emotional changes of motherhood, there are memory
changes as well. As in, you will have lapses in short-term memory.
I've heard it termed *mom brain, brain mush,* or *pregnancy brain.*
I like the term *Jell-O brain.* Interestingly, the brain is sort of the
consistency of Jell-O, so pictures of Jell-O-mold brains really do
freak me out.

Expect to experience changes in how you think and remember
things after a baby. This may not stress you out if you are a "go with
the flow" type of person, and forgetting where you put the bottle you
need to clean doesn't matter to you. If you are the type of person who
likes to *know,* then be proactive about how you will address mommy

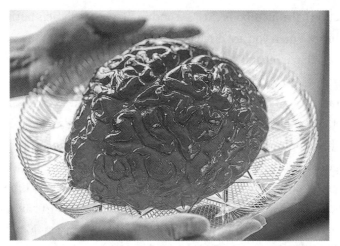

This is a brain made entirely of Jell-O. After you give birth it can feel that your brain is made of Jell-O. Rest assured it does not change into Jell-O—but how you think and remember things changes.   *Courtesy of Rich Brainerd*

brain. Develop systems for cleaning and storage, or make a lot of lists. My cellphone notes app is essentially my external brain, but you might have a more complex system of accounts.

A Hairy Situation

An annoying, embarrassing, and mentally taxing phenomenon of the postpartum period is hair loss. It doesn't happen immediately, but usually a few weeks to 3 months after birth it begins for many. It has a fancy name: postpartum telogen effluvium. I'm not even going to sound that out for you; just think postpartum hair loss. The name is a nod to the 3 phases of hair growth, the last being telogen, or the resting phase of hair as it sits on your head just looking pretty (hopefully, you like your hair). Like many conditions affecting women, research on this phenomenon is a little scarce. It is just something that happens, and we blame the hormones adjusting after birth. We then call it a day and live with it. Why do we do that?

In pregnancy, though, hair growth is really preserved. Increased levels of progesterone and estrogen (thanks almighty placenta) keep the hair happy. It not only grows faster, but there are reports that it might growth thicker. So, you have more luxurious hair. Then you give birth and, boom, estrogen and progesterone levels fluctuate, and with some time the hair sheds. For the record, your hair is always shedding, but generally each strand is on its own time schedule. But after pregnancy the hair has hung out for a while, and then all the hair strands decide to jump ship together. It's been estimated that at around 9 weeks after delivery, about a third of your hair is ready to shed—eek. The anterior hair line right around the forehead is most noticeable. Some women get bangs, not to reclaim their school-aged years, but to hide the tiny tufts of hair sporadically sprouting from their scalps. Not only does it fall out, the texture changes. My hair was much scragglier when it returned from its perfect pregnancy mane. This was also frustrating.

Your baby also experiences hormonal changes and loses their hair with you. So, there is solace in not being alone. And generally, babies develop true bald spots, which is also important because misery loves company, and you can be "baldish" together. Both of my children had a classic ring of hair loss on the back of their heads from sleeping on their back at night.

So, what to do about this? Dermatologists can help with different types of hair loss. Your primary care provider also might have suggestions or at least be a good listener. The mantra "hang in there, it gets better" is fitting for new moms in general and applies in this case as well because most women's hair seems to grow back, but it can take up to 15 months after giving birth. So think about cutting your hair (mom cut!), trying new styles, getting those bangs, or switching to a fancier shampoo. Do what you need to do for your hairdo.

Simply the Breast

No surprise that your chest will change. After delivery, your body will make milk whether you want to use it to feed your baby or not. We are going to get into breastfeeding in Chapter 6, but here we will talk about those breast changes. Additionally, if milk making is your thing, but for whatever reason your baby can't have the milk, there is the option to donate your milk to a public milk bank. For more information on donating your milk please use this QR code.

During pregnancy you might notice the first changes to the breast, areola, and nipple. The nipple darkens, presumably to become a bull's eye of sorts for a baby when they feed. The breasts become bigger and more tender. Mine looked particularly veiny as well. It might also surprise you that your breast tissue extends all the way into your arm pits, so you can feel the ducts enlarging there. I also felt there were more hairs around my nipple, which I imagined would tickle the baby's face during feeding, but really were probably just the result of more retained hair in pregnancy from hormonal changes. These changes to breasts occur so they will be able to start making and holding onto milk.

But it's not like there are geysers of milk shooting from both of your breasts immediately after delivery. Firstly, there is something to be said for mothers who overproduce. It's uncomfortable to make too much milk. Plus, having a strong letdown could drown your poor baby. So maybe it's for the best that your body isn't spraying milk right away. Full-on milk production starts anywhere from 3 to 5 days after you deliver. If you are directly feeding your newborn, or putting them on your chest to feed, this is when your nipple exam becomes essential. They (meaning some of the breastfeeding gurus) always talk about how it shouldn't hurt when you breastfeed. This is not true because pain is subjective and no one can tell you if you are in pain except for you. That and if it doesn't hurt the body, it can hurt the soul. In so many ways breastfeeding can feel like a spiritual experience, but let's get back to your body. Breastfeeding is uncomfortable early on; your nipple is sensitive and having someone suck on it is not exactly fun. But if you are experiencing stabbing or shooting pains that last throughout the feeding, this is a sign that you need to get checked out. The most common reason for pain with breastfeeding early on is the way in which the baby attaches to or latches onto the nipple. Also, if the nipple develops a lipstick appearance after feeds—meaning it's flattened on one side with a point on the top— that is another sign that the latch is bad. Nipples should never look like lipstick. In addition to shape, you want to make sure your nipple isn't cracked or bleeding; this can also be a sign of a suck that's taking in too much nipple and not enough areola.

Later on, breasts do best when the milk flows freely through them. That's why underwire bras or anything pushing on or restricting the breast is not recommended. For those with larger breasts, like this author, not wearing underwire can make you feel too loose. It was worth it to me to buy some nicer bras to get through breastfeeding and keep my breasts safe and supported. Sometimes, despite the best counseling on lactation and monitoring, your physical exam can still reveal issues with your breasts. A friend of mine developed something called a clogged duct. That's when there is an area in which the milk doesn't flow well and it sits in the breast. My friend started noticing this when she developed a white painful dot on her nipple called a milk bleb. This is when a nipple pore or duct becomes blocked right where the milk exits. Hot showers and picking at the painful nubbin helped. When a duct is blocked, the entire breast can feel tender or lumpy and sometimes gets a little red. As a result, it's at risk for infection, so making sure to watch for this and intervening with changes of clothes, massages, electric toothbrushes to the breast, and the like is very important. Continued breastfeeding through these challenges, like clogged milk ducts or mastitis, also can help with the flow.

After finishing breastfeeding, I saw changes on my breasts. I noticed more stretch marks on my breasts and both my cup size and band size increased. Some women report that their breasts go back to the prepregnancy measurements. This likely depends on your milk storage capacity and how long you breastfed. Sometimes though I blame age and gravity more than feeding my baby.

Can You Stomach This?

You carried that baby in your belly so your abdominal exam is going to be different from what it was before pregnancy. Aside from watching my belly expand and not realizing my baby bump was going to be unwieldy at 39 weeks' gestation, one thing that happened to me is something termed *linea nigra*, meaning literally black line. I had one that extended from my belly button down to my pelvis. Women report a lot of skin changes in pregnancy, but since we are talking about the postpartum period, I'm not going to list them all here. If you have any questions, make sure to contact your doctor for guidance. That said, my linea nigra stayed with me for several months postpartum. There are many myths surrounding the line, which about 80% of pregnant women develop in some form. Some people think it helps to point the baby toward the nipple (I would argue though it's not an arrow) while others think you can determine a baby's sex organs by the size or length of the line (you can't). Also, during pregnancy your belly button may go from an innie to an outie. This didn't happen to me, as my belly button is a dark cavern hiding a lint collection. My belly button does seem forever stretched though.

The stretch is the key factor to changes in your belly. You have a set of muscles that run on either side of your belly button and extend from your ribs all the way down to your pelvis. You might have heard of these abdominal muscles in a spin, Pilates, or yoga class: rectus abdominus. Sort of like the name of a dinosaur, likely a carnivorous one. These rectus abdominus muscles come together in the middle of the stomach on a piece of connective tissue. During an exam of the baby, you might see something called diastasis recti. Again, likely some sort of progeny of a *Tyrannosaurus rex*. Newborns have this because they don't need those big abdominal muscles to be developed, at least yet. They spend most of the day sleeping and moving their arms and legs in random patterns. Usually, by around 8 weeks the muscles start to tighten up, and by adulthood any traces of diastasis recti from infancy are long gone. That said, diastasis recti is common after pregnancy.

If you are pregnant more than 1 or 2 times, you are likely to have diastasis recti to some degree. I feel this condition is what prompted a close friend to get a tummy tuck. She didn't get a full "mommy makeover," which I learned refers to a tummy tuck and breast lift after delivery. You might need a little more time than that to recover. I naively thought a tummy tuck was just removing some old skin that was stretched out and hanging after being deflated postdelivery. It's a little more aggressive than that. The procedure involves sewing together your abdominal muscles—the rectus abdominus—that had gotten stretched or pulled apart after you delivered. This pulling apart is why many women feel their bodies are just hanging out after they deliver. I remember having a flat stomach in my 20s. Now, my stomach is large, especially on the bottom. I asked my father-in-law, a retired plastic surgeon, if he thought I had diastasis recti and should get a tummy tuck. As any good doctor making a diagnosis, he asked me to lie down so he could examine my abdominal muscles. Then, without warning, he essentially karate chopped me in the gut. Shoving the side of his hand into my belly to determine if he could forcefully feel the separation. I had my breath knocked out of me and my confidence shattered. Oh, this is why I couldn't return to the flat stomach of my youth, because I did have diastasis recti. That said, surgery is not the only solution—dedicated physical therapy and exercises can help strengthen the abdomen and return it to a state more like it was.

Pelvic Floor Tour

We are moving down to one area of the body that suffered a huge blow from pregnancy and delivery: the undercarriage. I like to call it that, in part because it's not something you ever really see. Much like the underside of a carriage, your pelvic floor will be abused and dirtied, and seeing the damage is difficult. A mirror can help you peer up there, but you will feel the effects of it. The initial weeks after you deliver is a good time to survey how your body has changed.

Remember, you need time and space to heal. Whether you have a surgical incision right above your pelvis or tears throughout your vagina, these areas need to heal. After a few weeks postpartum, you might see some nagging changes that were precipitated by the delivery and can linger for a long time.

One of my main problems is peeing myself unexpectedly. In no scenario is peeing yourself ok. Some birth parents might say, "Well everyone pees themselves after having a baby, that's totally normal." I haven't ever felt it's normal to urinate on myself. I'll be laughing at a joke, or sneezing, or jumping rope and a little bit of urine will escape my urethra. If I'm not in public, I'll sort of accept it grudgingly. If I am with other people, I'll ditch the fun-loving party that got me belly laughing, clean myself up, and vow to clench my Kegels tightly the next time I want to have fun. After my third baby I started wearing those superthin pads that are made for light period flow, but I think they should be specifically marketed for postpartum tinkle.

Again, you can tighten up this area with exercise before and after giving birth. Some physical therapists specialize in helping rehabilitate the undercarriage after the bumpy ride of birth. Seek out insurance coverage for this and a person who really knows what exercises will help.

Let's also talk about the vagina. If you gave birth through it, it's been through it. If you gave birth via a surgical c-section, the vagina can still feel the hormonal twists and turns of the postpartum period. Many birth parents won't have their periods after they deliver. Yay! But one hormone they might lack when they aren't cycling is estrogen. Not having estrogen can make the vagina feel, well, dry. Like desert dry. This is a time when your sex drive is probably on cruise control or worse, it's parked at a rest stop. A dry vagina can also be uncomfortable, and during sex it can be painful. Talk to your doctor about whether you need medication to help the vagina rejuvenate.

Feet

Do you know what they say about a birth parent with big feet? They probably just had a baby. Seriously. Your feet can stretch and get bigger, and you may end up a whole shoe size larger than you were before having your baby. So, hopefully you have a friend to whom you can pass down all those fun flat and funky heels you wore before you gave birth. Time to size up and step up into your changed physical and emotional role as a parent.

Chapter 5

Testing 1, 2, 3

*T*he postpartum experience in the nursery can be rough, and multiple interruptions to check on the health of mom and baby leave
little downtime to just enjoy the experience of having a healthy
newborn. To not add to the multiple interruptions to dyadic or couplet
care with birth parent and baby we round in a conference room.

On this day, we got to a patient I'll call Lila. I listened attentively
as we discussed her routine care as a healthy newborn. Then it came:
the gut punch. The parents refused vitamin K and the hepatitis B
vaccine. I get a visceral reaction to hearing these refusals, and after
years of working in the nursery that hasn't changed. A pit forms in my
stomach, and I start thinking how we failed this family. I am crying as
I write about it. I can't believe we have gotten to a point in the world
where lifesaving interventions are turned away with confidence. Interventions that can help children live healthy, safe lives are considered
hazardous and unnecessary because false information has found a
footing in medicine.

I've had to adopt a thick skin when someone refuses a vaccine.
Years and years of misinformation (inaccurate information) and
even disinformation (false information deliberately spread) about the
incredible benefits of vaccines have worn immunity in children thinner and thinner. Outbreaks of illnesses like measles and pertussis have
begun to spread and disrupt some communities. Still, many would
like to turn to the misinformation, saying given the choice they would
rather put their child through a harrowing illness and risk infecting

others than allow for a vaccine. It feels awful not helping people to see the advantages of protecting their children and their communities from preventable infections. And there are whole books about the overwhelming benefit of vaccines...but to not get a vitamin shot? I struggle more with the sadness of this because the downsides of getting a vitamin shot are...well, almost nonexistent. Vitamin K is essential in preventing devastating bleeds in babies—so why not get it?

My mind flashes to 2 things. The first is what the family must think about medicine. Here they are delivering in a hospital and the very routine vitamins we recommend for every baby because of the overwhelming evidence they're lifesaving...are deliberately tossed aside. They are not trusted, and that distrust is palpable. It translates to a lack of trust in the medical system, a belief the system is flawed and the people in it (eg, pediatricians and neonatologists like me) are complicit in its failures. Parents have told me that since I've been trained by the system, I can't even see its flaws. You might think that's paranoid, but I don't. I think it's a symptom of the system's failure in the United States to treat so many people as human. I've had that happen, as insurance companies refused to cover emergency treatments for my own child. It makes me really question the health care system I work in so closely. So, while I was trained in it, I think there is a lot of room for improvement. And then there is this family, forced to engage in medical care they don't have faith in and wanting to take back some control and humanity. I can't tell you how brave I think that is. Confounding, because they trusted the system enough to deliver in it, but also courageous as they try to make loving choices for their infant while bombarded with increasing mis- and disinformation making decision-making difficult when it should be routine and easy. We can and must do better to earn people's trust, because trust is never something that is just given—it is deserved and built.

This leads me to my second thought—how can I help Lila? How do I communicate effectively and teach and earn that trust? A lot of times

I can persuade parents to give vitamin K to baby boys. The promise of a circumcision in the hospital pushes them to protect their baby for the procedure. Vitamin K is essential in preventing hemorrhagic disease or uncontrolled bleeding in a newborn. This bleeding—striking generally at several weeks after birth—was more common before we made sure babies received vitamin K. However, like so many preventable diseases, it's on the rise because preventive medicine is under attack. Generally we as adults get vitamin K from our diet and our gut bacteria churning it out. (A reminder that not all bacteria are bad.) Babies only drink milk and don't have developed gut bacteria in their intestines, so they don't produce vitamin K. If they are breastfed, they are even less likely to get vitamin K. Unfortunately, it's the parents who breastfeed who tend to want a more "natural" approach. Nature is a fickle beast and one that doesn't prioritize protecting babies, which is why we need to. Without vitamin K, at around 6 weeks after birth, babies are at risk for internal bleeding, which can drain major organs and most notably the brain. This bleeding is preventable with 1 shot of vitamin K. Just 1 shot. The same thing I have to try to convince Lila's parents how much she needs this vitamin.

I listened to Lila's family, hearing things I'd heard before.

"I don't see the point of giving it," the parent said. (There's a huge reason to. Preventing devastating bleeding.)

"I think it will cause them to be more jaundiced." (This was a new one for me, as vitamin K has no association with jaundice.)

"I don't want to do it just because everyone else does." (Everyone else does because it's safe and truly protects your baby from bleeding.)

"I've done my reading. I've made my decision." (What did you read? Did you check the sources? Have they seen babies die or become unable to live full lives because they were denied a vitamin that could protect their brain?) I don't want to scare you, and I don't want to fact-check your sources. I'm here for your baby and your family to educate and listen. There are families whose children suffered from not getting this shot.

For more information on real-life stories about babies and vitamin K please use this QR code.

I told the family I knew we disagreed, but I wanted to keep the lines of communication open. I complimented them for being so thoughtful about their baby, for showing so much love in wanting the best for her. I told them I wished I could build a bridge between us. That I could prove to them I wanted what's best for her too, and this wasn't just me trying to doctor them—it was me caring for them. I hope they know I tried to help Lila. They don't know I am crying for her now. While my brain doesn't bleed, my heart does. People think we leave the hospital and our patients behind and wash our hands of them at the end of the day—this is not true. I spent time when Lila was discharged worrying—as I do for all families that refuse this shot— that she might have a bleed and or lose her ability to do what typical children can do. I'm sad her family didn't trust medical advice, that they felt wronged by it. That they have turned to sources that are not looking to protect and truly educate them. How did we get here as a society—that we can't even protect all our youngest members with vitamins to help them flourish? Lila, I want to do better for you. I won't give up. We can make this a better and more healing system for you. Stay safe little one.

There are always tears when a baby is born. So much emotion is packed into a busy delivery room brimming with the energy of new life. Even the labor and delivery nurses who have already delivered 5 babies on their shift have a twinkle in their eye when a new one is passed to them. Ideally, newborns spend the first hour of their lives with their birth parent; they then are treated with some initial interventions meant to secure a healthy start. This gives them the best chance for healthy bonding with you later. Let's review.

Eyes and Thighs: Delivery of Eye Goop and Vitamin K

Infants often receive 2 things in the delivery room: erythromycin eye ointment and vitamin K. Let's start with the eye ointment. Birth parents receiving good prenatal care will be tested for infectious diseases including gonorrhea and chlamydia. Both types of bacteria can hang out in the vagina and spread to the baby. Gonorrhea (and to a lesser extent chlamydia) is notorious for a type of goopy eye infection that can really mess with the eyes of tiny babies whose immune systems are not so good. Thus, we give them eye ointment to protect them. However, if a parent has had good prenatal care and testing, the eye ointment likely isn't doing much, and I don't squabble with families who really don't want it done. I work in a state that doesn't legally require you give this ointment. There are some where it is illegal not to give this eye goop. If you are in a state that requires it, you will be given it. The American Academy of Pediatrics (AAP) does want states to reevaluate this, as there are more important interventions for new babies we know make a big difference for them.

Vitamin K is one of those things. This is a vitamin I'll go to the mat for. While vitamin K is, as its name implies, a vitamin, it has somehow begun to earn a reputation as something more sinister. Some crazy compound pushed onto unsuspecting newborns. It has become fashionable to reject this shot as it symbolizes the medical-industrial complex and isn't "natural" or necessary.

I fully endorse questioning and changing the behemoth of the health care system I work in. I applaud efforts to make things better. I love hearing from patients about new ideas and alternative methods so I can understand what they do and so we can work together to make things better. But to refuse vitamin K? This vitamin is not a profit-driven cash cow thrust upon families to suck from the teat of insurance companies and garner millions of dollars by poking the legs of unsuspecting babies. Vitamin K is an essential vitamin that newborns lack and administering it has saved the lives of countless babies. I say countless literally because we don't know exactly how many have been saved just by receiving the vitamin.

Vitamin K is a helper. It is a key ingredient in helping the body form blood clots and prevent bleeding. Before we knew how critical this vitamin was at 6 weeks after birth, infants would die from bleeding out of every part of their body. While I was on a medical rotation in Ghana, one mother brought her baby to the hospital. She had delivered in a rural section of the country and the baby had not received vitamin K, as it was not available. The result was devastating and I do not want to describe it to you here except to use the word gruesome. I had never seen anything like it, but the Ghanaian attending had. "That's hemorrhage disease of the newborn," he said, sadly but knowingly, with the face of someone less horrified because he'd seen this before. I haven't just seen a baby with this condition in the Ghanaian countryside. I met a well-to-do Los Angeles couple sobbing at the side of their baby's bedside when I was a resident. I didn't know how to respond to their sadness, as I was still learning how to approach families devastated by this tragedy. Their baby, previously healthy and interactive, had a brain bleed at a few weeks of age. It left the baby nearly comatose. The culprit? The same hemorrhagic disease of the newborn I had seen in Ghana. They had refused vitamin K not because of a lack of access, but because they felt it wasn't necessary. The mother looked in my eyes and asked me, "Could this have been prevented if I gave the vitamin K shot?" I looked down at the floor and mumbled yes. We cried together.

If you want a nontraditional birth and to buck the confines of our often chaotic and confusing medical world, that's fine. If you want to do research and try to pick the perfect birth plan, that's also wonderful and let's talk about it (but be prepared for the experience to not meet all your expectations). If you want to skip the vitamin K shot—don't. Infants just don't make vitamin K the way we do. Our guts are filled with bacteria that work with us to make this vitamin, and we can choose foods that help supplement it in our adult diets. Newborns don't yet have a gut colonized by the bacteria needed to create this vitamin, and they don't eat anything but milk. This shot was developed in response to the anguish experienced by families over the loss of a baby they had held and loved for several weeks. Bleeding in the brain from vitamin K deficiency, which is also known as a stroke, can happen. Statistics show real people are experiencing this preventable complication and it is shattering. It robs you of joy, of the previously healthy baby you held right after delivery. Bleeding in the brain from vitamin K deficiency is not common.

Again, I'm not asking you to get vitamin K because it lines my pockets or because I've been brainwashed by the medical system into thinking there is one way of doing things and vitamin K is the way. I'm asking you because *I do not* want to be sitting in the neonatal intensive care unit (NICU) with you as you cry next to your precious child. *I do not* want you to ask me if what happened was preventable because *I do not* want to have to tell you it could have been. I want you to help your new baby grow to their fullest potential, and I know that if they don't receive the vitamin K shot, there is a real possibility they won't. It's a small one but made small because vitamin K is so routine. As more families rely on misinformation to justify not giving it, I'm worried that an increasing number of families will see this horrible and devastating disease. *I do not* want you to realize the importance of vitamins after the fact, while your baby's life hangs in the balance. And *I do not* want this to alter the course of your life, for you to be another story on the Centers for Disease Control and Prevention website about these incredibly awful bleeds. *I want* you to bond with your baby, to build a relationship without worry. I want that for you.

I'm not asking you to get the vitamin K shot for the good of humanity or your community. I'm asking you to do it for your baby, no one else but them. I know you can't trust all the noise out there in infant care, but the signal here is clear—this is a potentially lifesaving injection and one you are going to want your baby to get. It is a simple, inexpensive miracle of modern medicine. An experience your baby and you won't even remember—a shot in the thigh that can save you from untold heartache.

You might be thinking she keeps saying a shot, I'll give vitamin K but I'll just make the baby take it by mouth to spare them an injection. I cannot recommend you give vitamin K this way. Remember the baby's gut is immature, so will it absorb all the vitamin K? We don't know. Additionally, we don't know the appropriate amount to give, or for how long to give it. And have you tried to give your baby an oral medication? If you have you know it can be challenging, and half of it can wind up outside of their mouth. The most effective way to make sure your baby receives the right amount of vitamin K is with a shot. Give them that shot to help prevent bleeding issues during the weeks you should be bonding.

Baby's Routine Screens

I See You PKU

The exam is done. You have a typical baby with their own physical quirks. I saw that little ear pit they have and you have one too. Aside from looking at the baby's body, we perform other testing to assess their physiology, or how the body functions. Little noninvasive (aka not very painful or long) tests to help us make sure the healthy baby we see on the outside is set up for success through and through. The first test being the PKU.

The acronym PKU stands for painfully krafted utility. Ok, that's not true, though it does involve a needle and heel sticks, which babies don't love. It stands for phenylketonuria (fen-el-keto-yuri-a), a metabolic condition in which the body can't break down certain types of protein (namely, phenylalanine). So a toxic buildup of the protein is left in your body, which can cause you to get sick or worse if it's not recognized.

Why am I telling you about PKU? It's not because I think your baby will have it, it's because it was the very first test included in something referred to as *PKU or newborn screening.* It is a part of the testing done in newborns at around 24 hours old. The PKU or newborn screen consists of taking a little bit of blood from the heel of the baby and sending it off to a state lab to test for various genetic, metabolic, and hormonal conditions. Not all newborn screens are created equal, because every state tests for a different panel of conditions. Where you deliver will determine the extent of your newborn screen.

I work primarily in Pennsylvania, and we test for something called G6PD deficiency, or glucose-6-phosphate dehydrogenase deficiency. This is an enzyme deficiency that can affect how red blood cells function. The state neighboring mine—New Jersey—doesn't test for that. You don't have to move to a state with more expansive screening, but you can find out what screening is done in your state and then ask your pediatrician if you are worried about something your state doesn't screen for. At the time of writing, Missouri screened for the most conditions (77), while North Dakota screened for the fewest (32). Most items on the screen are relatively rare, but if caught early can be life changing. For example, it's good to know if a baby has PKU because you can alter the proteins they eat starting in infancy and help them achieve normal growth and intelligence without any of the nasty developments of PKU. Pretty cool, right? All from a few drops of blood; that's exciting science.

For more information on the newborn screening requirements for the state you live in please use this QR code.

Critical Congenital Heart Disease (CCHD) Checks for Baby

Next is what I refer to as the oxygen test. It doesn't involve giving oxygen, but it does involve something called a pulse oximeter or pulse ox. Pulse oximeter use became pretty widespread during the COVID-19 pandemic; my parents now have a pulse ox in their medicine cabinet that they slap on whenever they have a runny nose to test their oxygen levels. They are in their 70s so their medical concerns don't quite fit the age range of this book (of note, they are still building a relationship with me, so that part fits).

You can also buy a pulse ox for your baby at home. Not something I recommend but something companies would love to sell you on. Hospitals have fancier pulse oximeters that are time and technology tested to use in infants. Companies have altered that technology and marketed it as a way to keep babies safe at home. However, there is no evidence to suggest these devices are a good safety tool. There is no replacement for a family checking in on their infant at night. Infants are not programmed to sleep through the night (more on this in Chapter 7), and checking in on them is so important. Additionally, given there is no scientific testing routinely done on these commercial machines, when your pediatrician reviews the data with you, they might not be familiar with the pulse ox from the company you chose and how to interpret its data. False alarms can also happen, so when the machines do pick up events at home, there isn't a way to verify their severity. This is something all parents should be mindful of; technology can be a wonderful thing, but it cannot replace you as your baby's number 1.

Back to using a pulse oximeter in the hospital. The pulse ox screen is called the critical congenital heart disease screen, or CCHD screen. People often think of oxygen as being a lung thing, but the heart (if you remember from our discussion of the physical exam in chapter 4) is the organ responsible for taking that oxygen-rich blood and pumping it out to the body. Without the heart, the work of the lungs could not be appreciated by organs like the kidney or body parts like the tips of your toes. Checking the pulse ox in a newborn gives a sense of how the lungs are taking in oxygen, as well as how the heart is pumping it out. When you think of the heart as just a large pump, it's hard not to use plumbing analogies, so that's how I'll describe this test.

If you want water to come out of your bathroom sink, the faucet needs to be attached to plumping that connects to a water source. If you want to get that oxygen-rich blood from the lungs and heart (aka the internal pipes and tubing you can't see) to the body (aka the faucet), there can be no leaks in the system (no one likes water damage in their house) and no other place to which the blood can travel outside of your plumbing system. Also, the heart isn't very smart. It just beats; it doesn't think about where the blood is going but just sends it forth into the body with some major metronome vibes. The blood loves to follow the path of least resistance. If a baby's heart isn't configured correctly, or the pipes aren't connected the right way, the blood is going to flow where there is nothing obstructing its path. That might mean that some parts of your body aren't going to receive the oxygen they need. Ideally, the same oxygen is in all parts of the body at the same time. But if the faucet isn't working or the pipes are leaky, oxygen is not going to go where it needs to go.

The CCHD screen consists of one pulse oximeter placed on the right hand and another on the left leg to ensure the oxygen quality of the blood is the same in both places; greater than 95% is considered normal. If a baby fails the test, more investigation is needed into how the heart is pumping blood to the body. Usually, an echocardiogram is obtained to get a picture of the heart and see where the plumbing issue might lie.

Hearing Screen Machine

Being deaf or hard of hearing isn't as uncommon as you might think. About 1 to 3 in 1,000 newborns may have significant hearing loss at birth. In the 1990s, organizations like the AAP started to recommend universal hearing screens in infants to detect hearing impairments early on and be able to provide resources to families to help with communication and ultimately how that baby will connect with caregivers and the world.

One of the reasons it's nice to deliver in a hospital is that it has the machinery needed to perform the hearing screen in a newborn. Some pediatricians also offer this screening in their pediatric offices so make sure to ask. Making an appointment with a hearing specialist or an audiologist might be more challenging, as they might not be equipped to evaluate infants or have a long waiting list for appointments.

So how is this hearing screen done? Depending on what machine is used by your hospital and how quiet all the rooms are, the test can be performed in your hospital room or the infant might be taken back to the nursery for the screen. Headphones or earmuff-looking contraptions are put over the baby's ears. Generally, a sensor is also placed on the head or forehead of the baby. These are meant to measure 2 things: 1) how well the brain interprets sound or neurologic hearing and 2) hairs and membranes in the ear that help move sound around; this is referred to as the conductive portion of hearing. The sensors are meant to look at brain activity. Much like the heart, which puts out electrical impulses to beat, the brain also puts out electrical signals for the neurons to communicate with each other. The hearing screen machine is meant to pick up on these signals and on the sensory impulses to from the ear, which is the sensory-neurologic or sensorineural part of hearing.

The ideal environment to perform this screen is a quiet room without any background noise. The baby should be asleep, so not crying, sucking on a bottle or pacifier, or moving around. The conditions I outlined are Anne Geddes ideal. We have special technicians in the nursery who really try to create these conditions and sometimes succeed. We want babies to be able to "pass" in both ears. When they don't pass in both ears at the same time, we can't count the screen as a pass. If your newborn does not pass the hearing screening, we call it a "refer," meaning the infant needs more formal hearing evaluation outside the hospital with a specialist in audiology.

Having your baby fail a hearing screen can be emotional; you will then wonder if they have trouble hearing or are hard of hearing. If that's the case, it's good to know early on and you should feel empowered to have this information. Often, though, there won't be a true issue with their hearing, but there might be an issue with the machine or how well the baby tolerated the procedure. That's why most hospitals give babies at least 2 chances to pass the screen. If your baby does refer, many states recommend testing for a virus called *cytomegalovirus*, or CMV. CMV is a common virus that infects people of all ages. Many adults in the United States have been infected with CMV—I know I was because I underwent CMV testing along with my fertility testing in my third pregnancy. Once you have CMV, it can hang out in the body forever. It is possible though that pregnant parents often are not screened for CMV because so many people would test positive, and many times they don't need treatment, and neither will their baby. It is possible, though, that pregnant people can pass CMV to their baby, and this is called congenital CMV. We think people who become infected with CMV during pregnancy have the highest risk of passing it on to their baby. In the United States, it is thought that about 200 infants are born annually with CMV, but they don't show signs of infection at birth. Of those 200 infants, around 1 in 5 or 40 of them could go on to develop longer-term health issues including hearing loss. That's why more states want babies tested for CMV if they don't pass their hearing screen. We test by taking either a little bit of saliva or urine, so it's not painful. If an infant does have CMV after being referred on their hearing screen discussing treatment with your pediatrician is important.

Most infants pass their newborn hearing screen; however, if yours doesn't, don't despair. Follow these steps:

- Follow up with your pediatrician.
- Get a referral for your baby to see an audiologist.
- Complete a CMV test.

Be proactive in making sure your infant has the best possible hearing development. Hearing screening doesn't stop at birth; it only begins there. Make sure to ask your pediatrician about your baby's hearing, language development, and speech at your baby's well-child visits and as they grow.

It Was all Yellow

Jaundice (jawn-dis...who dis? Jawn dis? For my Philadelphians out there, I know you will appreciate this pronunciation jawn; for everyone else, if you look it up you'll get my jawn) is something all babies experience. It's what we call physiologic and not pathologic (or bad). What is jaundice? It's the yellow discoloration of the skin and eyes that a baby can develop, generally in the first few days after delivery. Why does this happen? There are 3 main reasons.

The first is that babies' red blood cells—the cells that make that beautiful blood color—don't live as long as adult red blood cells. They break down more quickly and release something called bilirubin into the bloodstream. That bilirubin is yellow and it contributes to the color of your infant's poop and pee.

A second reason why bilirubin levels get high is the liver is supposed to help the body process it. However, the liver of infants is immature and can't quite do the job, especially in those first few days after birth. So, more bilirubin in the bloodstream with less ability to break it down results in jaundice. Lastly, if you breastfeed, your infant is likely to be jaundiced and for a longer time. We are not 100% sure why, but early on it could do with babies taking small volumes of milk and being a little dehydrated. Outside of the first week after birth we think it has to do with how the body breaks down breast milk.

While you might have heard of jaundice before or know a friend or family member whose baby needed to be treated for it, don't get anxious about it. I'm here to tell you it's not all bad. We believe bilirubin has antioxidant properties, so there is probably some evolutionary reason why it becomes high in newborns. Doctors like to say that jaundice in a baby is always physiologic, meaning it's a typical body thing. Listen, though, there is something to be said for too much of a "good thing," and if bilirubin levels get too high, the bilirubin can cross into the brain and damage it. This brain injury (called kernicterus) is exceedingly rare in countries like the United States that check bilirubin levels in newborns and make sure infants can get treatment if the bilirubin level gets too high.

Some infants are at greater risk of developing jaundice than others. Differing blood types between the birth parent and the baby can cause jaundice. If a baby isn't eating well, dehydration can cause jaundice because poop (and to a lesser extent pee) are the best ways to get bilirubin levels down. Different types of genetic conditions can also cause jaundice if they cause red blood cells to break down quicker (some of these conditions are tested for on the PKU, or the newborn screen).

As I said earlier, management of jaundice causes stress for many families. Treatment for it touches on the one thing that can bring up so much anxiety for families—feeding your baby. Remember, babies who are breastfed are more likely to be jaundiced. It's common, especially in first-time parents, that the milk supply won't come in for around 3 to 5 days. Something like jaundice can make them feel as if they are failing at breastfeeding. For a baby with a high bilirubin level, or jaundice, pumping is recommended (we will go more into this in Chapter 6, but pumping helps the milk supply come in faster, and you can feed the extra breast milk you pump to baby), or supplementation with donor human milk or formula may be offered to help because they aren't eating enough. It's hard to juggle this constant need to feed with the need for more blood checks, more monitoring, and possibly a longer hospital stay for treatment of the high bilirubin level. It should come as no surprise that just as a person's milk comes in at about days 3 to 5, that's also when the bilirubin level usually peaks. Given most families leave the hospital before the third day after birth, jaundice can follow them around for the first week. If one of the pediatric health care professionals helping to take care of your baby tells you they are worried your infant might need treatment for jaundice, ask them these questions:

1. How quickly is my baby's bilirubin level rising? The rate of rise matters.
2. When do you think it might reach the level needed for treatment? They should be able to show you a curve.
3. Do you offer any treatments at home, or only in the hospital?
4. Do you recommend I supplement with more milk to help with this jaundice? Can we go over what types of milk you have here or how I might pump?

Then ask yourself:

1. Will it stress me out to be chasing these bilirubin levels when I go home?
2. Can I stay in the hospital longer? Do I need to go home and am I ok with coming back for more monitoring or if my baby needs treatment?

The treatment for jaundice is phototherapy. Phototherapy involves use of an intense blue light, whose light waves can penetrate the skin and help the body eliminate (through pee) the bilirubin. It is extraordinarily effective and almost all infants respond beautifully to it. There are a few drawbacks to this kind of therapy. First, the baby has to be unwrapped so the skin is exposed, and newborns don't like this. Next, they need to wear glasses to protect their eyes, and oftentimes they fall off. The amount of time under these lights counts, so planning for breaks to feed and snuggle can be challenging. Unfortunately, phototherapy is usually only done in hospitals, but at-home treatment is becoming more widely accepted.

Screening bilirubin levels generally occurs at 12 to 24 hours after birth, and then repeated checks are dictated by the initial levels and how quickly they rise over time (if levels fall, the newborn is in the clear). To prepare yourself for the emotional roller coaster of jaundice management, it's helpful to ask yourself the following: Has anyone in your family had jaundice? Is the birth parent's blood type O (they are more likely to make antibodies against baby blood cells) or is there a negative sign at the end of their blood type? Does the birth parent have any known antibodies against red blood cells? And know that jaundice does require close watching of feeds, so if your baby has it, be prepared to supplement feeds, whether it be with pumping, donor human milk (if you have access to it), or formula. Most jaundice issues resolve in the first week after birth, so this is generally a short-term problem with no long-term follow-up.

To Vaccinate Is Great: Big Bad Hepatitis B Alongside RSV

Let's start by talking about your baby's first vaccines and the viruses they help protect the body from. Think of vaccines as presenting a unique opportunity to train your baby's body. They are an instruction manual or a guide for the baby's developing immune system—particularly the hepatitis B vaccine. The immunization against respiratory syncytial virus (RSV) is a little different. The shot actually provides antibodies or immunity to the baby right away. So, instead of the immune system learning about viruses—something called active immunity in which the immune system has to get up to speed on how to make antibodies against diseases—the RSV inoculation gives the newborn the antibodies they need. This is called passive immunity. Let's learn a little bit about these diseases.

Big Bad Hepatitis B

First, the wild world of hepatitis. "Hepa" is Greek for liver and any "itis" is an inflammation. These are viruses that cause inflammation or disease in the liver. When you learn about hepatitis it's an alphabet soup of viral names. Hepatitis A, B, C, D, and E can cause infections in people. To remember the different types of hepatitis in medical school, I learned catchy phrases to jog my memory better than the rote memorization of Greek words. The moniker "Big Bad Hepatitis B" has really worked for me. Because hepatitis B is arguably the worst type of hepatitis to get; it destroys the liver and promotes cancer. The third leading type of cancer? Liver cancer. And around half or maybe more of those cancers are caused by hepatitis B. It doesn't infect you and give you cancer in a few days or weeks. It plays the long game. Most people don't know they are infected until it's too late. Until the liver begins to fail, calling out, "Hey, this virus is overwhelming me. I have been fighting it for years, but I can't anymore." Before the introduction of the vaccine, entire families developed liver problems and cancer, and died of them, without knowing hepatitis B was to blame. These were not families in which everyone was an intravenous substance user or sleeping around. Hepatitis B is great at infecting people, even from tiny drops of blood. Just because you have a chronic disease caused by a virus doesn't mean you weren't careful or did something wrong; viruses are equal opportunity offenders. They love to spread, and they find ways to do it despite your best efforts. You can never be too careful about contracting Big Bad Hepatitis B, because it's always looking to find you.

Big Bad Hepatitis B likes to and is good at spreading in casual, undetected ways. It's spread by contact with blood but, remember, that once you have children you are exchanging bodily fluids as part of your parenting. What makes hepatitis B a great viral scourge is that just a tiny drop of blood can contain a lot of the virus. How might you get into contact with blood (yuck) and not know it? Let's say your child is at a sleepover and forgot their toothbrush so they use their friend's. Little bits of blood could be scraped up from their friend's gums and transferred into your child's mouth. Or maybe you are doing baby-led weaning and, much like a mother bird, you decide to help chew your baby's food and spit it out for them. Even if you are going to regularly scheduled dental visits, these rituals could be a potential exposure. Or maybe you are in the shower, and you use someone else's razor assuming the razor looks clean. But with any little microtears in the skin, tiny unseen droplets of blood can make it into your system, and it only takes that tiny bit of blood to infect you with hepatitis B. It's that good.

Many birth parents might think that since they were tested for hepatitis B and didn't have it, their baby won't get it. True, it's unlikely they will get it from you at delivery, or when they use your sore, torn-up nipples to breastfeed in the first few weeks. But you only know about your hepatitis status in the moment you got tested during pregnancy, not after. Also, people in the community don't routinely get tested for hepatitis B. I remember when my friend told me her mother had hepatitis B and found out at around age 65. My friend was shocked, and her mother's liver was already showing signs of wear and tear. She couldn't believe her mother, a woman in her 60s whose most exciting recreational activity was yoga outdoors, could have liver damage from a virus she associated with mischievous deeds. So even if you don't have hepatitis B at the time of your delivery, grandma or grandpa might. Or the babysitter could. Or your favorite uncle who is coming over for the holidays. Maybe even your partner who didn't undergo laboratory testing during your pregnancy.

Listen, I'm kind of scaring myself as I write this and that isn't my intention. But there is no other way to describe Big Bad Hepatitis B except to say it's an amazing, super agile virus. Just know that even if you are trying to be as careful as you possibly can, there is no "careful enough" with hepatitis B. With fewer people getting vaccinated, this virus will take advantage of a wane in our defenses to spread as best it can. It has a B in the name, but it's an A+ virus in terms of spread.

Knowing you can't be too careful, and there are many things you already worry about as a parent, you should then protect your baby when you can. Infants are advised to get the hepatitis B vaccine in the first 24 hours after birth. This is the first of many vaccinations for the baby. Your thoughts about vaccines before and after delivery are the foundation for how you will view them throughout your child's life, and your understanding of why vaccines work matters. Vaccines make everyone healthier; they are an amazing way to protect your community. Your community could be your immediate family, or your support network, or your whole city or town. By getting yourself and your infant vaccinated, you are protecting others. Not everyone has reliable access to health care, so ensuring you get vaccinated when you can and on a schedule helps protect those who can't easily get vaccinated. In other words, take your access to vaccination seriously when you can get it.

The most important reason to have your baby vaccinated for hepatitis B is that you want to build a long, healthy relationship with them. If an infant or a young child contracts hepatitis B, their chance of developing chronic liver disease is close to 100%. And remember that hepatitis B is a main cause of liver cancer, so getting this vaccine helps prevent a type of cancer. No one ever told me that in medical school, and I think it's important to know the power of this 1 shot. It acts as a way for your infant's body to study the virus before it gets infected. That way, if and when your baby's immune system comes into contact with hepatitis B, it can say, "Hum, I've read about this, I know what to do." And the baby's amazing little body can prevent infection so they can grow and thrive by your side.

Ruthless RSV

I receive a lot of texts about sick babies from my friends and family. I'll share 2 with you, both from before we had a vaccine for this illness.

TEXT CONVERSATION 1

Friend 1: "I just need someone to talk to; we had such a rough night. My baby boy has RSV. Our pediatrician tested him and now we are having to go to the office what feels like every day. Lots of crying, he is inconsolable. We keep doing nose suctioning and offering the boob. He is doing shorter nursing sessions so he's on the boob a lot. He is working hard on getting the congestion out. Lots of barking coughs, which is sad to hear but I think he's getting the mucus out. We haven't put him down, I'm just afraid I'll miss something."

At just 6 weeks old, this baby was not hospitalized, but the effort to keep him home was overwhelming. RSV made this family exhausted, worried, and at their wits' end for 2 weeks. I think the fact they kept their baby out of the hospital is heroic and admirable. Not all families are as lucky; consider text conversation 2. Our chat consisted of her explaining that the baby got RSV from their sibling, was doing very poorly, went to the emergency room, was intubated, and had to go to the pediatric intensive care unit (PICU) because there was no room in the NICU given the number of sick babies.

TEXT CONVERSATION 2

Friend 2: "My baby is now admitted to the PICU with RSV. I don't know what to do."

Me: "Hey. I'm so sorry to hear your baby is hospitalized for RSV. Want to chat on the phone?"

Friend 2 (a day later): "Hey. The baby is doing something that the doctor on the other night is puzzled by and I'm curious if you see more in the NICU. They are weaning their ventilator settings down, but they don't see a path to extubating them. Their respiratory rate is high since they made changes early in the shift. They are not really sure why her respiratory rate is so elevated."

I was pretty sure her lungs were still healing from the RSV. Knowing when to take a breathing tube out of a sick baby is always a difficult decision. We don't want to have to place the tube back in; we want them to be getting better. While most babies do improve from day to day, RSV is a virus that causes a lot of secretions that block the airway. So the recovery can be slow, weeks at a minimum. We never had a good vaccine or immunization for this virus until late in 2023. It's time we use it. Because these aren't the only texts I received about RSV, and parents should not be worried about how mechanical ventilators work when they should be bonding with baby.

RSV is a virus that can infect anyone but tends to make infants and older adults very sick. It is a respiratory virus, as the name suggests, so it's spread by coughing and sneezing and getting viral particles stuck in the eyes, nose, or mouth. It is a particularly sticky bug and can live on hard surfaces for a few hours; it also lives on soft surfaces but for a shorter amount of time. This virus is everywhere. By the time your child turns 2 years old, they have probably had it, and hopefully it was just a mild cold. But certain groups of people can get really sick from RSV; these include babies, especially those born prematurely, anyone with a weakened immune system, and people with heart conditions.

Now, there is a preventative medicine called nirsevimab that can be given to any infant to help them from getting sick with RSV. Note, they can still contract RSV, but this medication can prevent them from getting super sick. Nirsevimab is different from the hepatitis B vaccine in that it's not an instruction manual for the body. To illustrate, instead of going to Ikea and telling your immune system to make the coffee table on its own with all the proper pieces, this vaccine is like opting for white glove service—the coffee table is already assembled and delivered to your living room in one piece.

Nirsevimab is a monoclonal antibody, a protein made to neutralize infection in the body, and this one is specific to blocking RSV from harming your baby. It should be given within the first 7 days after birth, ideally shortly after birth, to protect the baby when they leave the hospital. Your birth hospital may be able to offer it to you. This is not the first antibody we've had to help prevent severe RSV infection in babies. You might have heard of palivizumab, especially

if you've had a preterm baby, one with heart disease, or one with some reason to be immunocompromised. Palivizumab wasn't for all babies, though, in part because of the cost (about $1,500 to $2,000 a shot) and in
part because it needed to be dosed every month throughout RSV season. So that was around 5 to 6 shots per baby. What's nice about nirsevimab is that it only costs around $500, so there is the hope that all insurance companies will cover this lifesaving treatment.

You'd rather get this antibody for your baby than have them get straight-up RSV. I say this knowing and hoping I might be out of a job, because I admit so many babies with RSV in cold and flu season into the hospital, but I don't want your baby to be one of them.

As doctors and nurses we do everything we can to help make sure babies get home healthy and stay that way during the newborn phase. There is only so much support we can provide you in the hospital. So, let's get you home and talk about what it's like to be with baby at your bedside rather than in the hospital.

Chapter 6

Finding Your Milk Way

I recognize not all families are cisgender and heteronormative. Chest or body feeding and human milk are more inclusive terms. However, I will use the terms breastfeeding and breast milk given their prevalence in scientific literature and my own experience. At the same time I acknowledge these terms are not all-encompassing.

W ith my first baby, breastfeeding went "well" during my brief 24-hour hospital stay. For me, breastfeeding "hurt" and anyone who tells you it doesn't is not telling the truth. (Note: I put a lot of apostrophes in this section because words like "well" and "hurt" are subjective.) My hurt could be your discomfort, or it could be the most pain you've ever felt. Feeding a baby makes you discover yourself and your boundaries in so many ways.) Though seriously, OUCH. The breast and nipples are sensitive parts of the body and getting repeatedly sucked on by a powerful insatiable vacuum leads to funky feelings—not all of them pleasant. After all, a woman's pain is meant to be endured, not discussed. Let's be honest: If men breastfed, there would be way more chatter about how much it hurts and way more forms of nipple protection. My nipples were tender and sore, but not cracked and bleeding, so I was one of the "lucky" ones. Also, the blinding pain from the intense cramping I had as my uterus contracted in response to nipple stimulation, totally normal. Yay! When I doubled over with latching, my postpartum nurse offered abundant reassurance. She helped me envision my empty, floppy uterus shrinking down to its original size and protecting me from postpartum blood loss. This was less comforting then I think she intended.

I didn't struggle with supply early on like so many women, who will outline their breastfeeding struggles. In fact, my early challenges were from engorgement and clogged ducts. My breasts became hard, hot, and alien appendages, swollen against my chest wall. Finding lactation support was difficult, and several calls of "Is this normal?" filled in the time between what seemed like constant feedings. After talking to some professional on the phone who gave instructions on hand massage and pumping, I called a good friend to vent with as I brushed my boob with an electric toothbrush hoping to open up some milk ducts. She said, "It's awful for the first 2 weeks; if you can get through those it will get better." That's still the best advice I've ever gotten about breastfeeding. Instead of, I must breastfeed for a year or more, I shifted to, let's see if I can breastfeed today. If I can today, maybe tomorrow too.

A pediatrician I visited in those early days commented that had it been the 1800s, I would have been a wet nurse, helping to breastfeed everyone in the community. I think he meant it as a compliment, but as I struggled to breastfeed my one baby, I had an overwhelming desire to firehose them in the face with my breast milk. Because my breasts would do just that—shoot streams of pressurized milk several feet when I squeezed them. I had to learn to feed my newborns lying down so they wouldn't gag on the milk that flew into their mouths, drowning them in nutrients.

Breastfeeding for me was desired, excruciating, humbling, and educating. As time went on, my goals changed, but my vigilance was constant. My wet nurse days ended abruptly with a return to work at around 3 months, and instead of overproducing, I shifted to barely making enough to cover the day. I made it to 10 months with my first child when I really wanted to make it to a year. With my second child, I made it to a full year. I credit making it to a year to the pandemic and the normalization of being home with my baby when I wasn't at work. I have come to realize, in a country that doesn't support new parents, any breastfeeding is an amazing achievement and a hard-won victory. With my third, again at 10 months I was thwarted by tongue-tie, poor weight gain, and supply issues. I didn't reach all my goals, and that's ok. It was still important for me to set them.

The powerful nutrient-giving placenta has completed its mission, and now you must nurture your new human. They need one form of nutrition: milk. Just as there are 2 ways a baby can exit a body, there are 2 main forms of nourishment for the baby: human milk or formula. Breastfeeding is a personal and cultural decision filled with emotion. Feelings and breastfeeding go together, which is why I will also talk about a birth parent's mental health in this chapter. So many lactating individuals almost intuitively tie their success as a parent to how and if they breastfeed. I want you to meet your goals for breastfeeding, whatever they are. I want you to have success and I want to encourage you to do your best. So I'll say this: How you feed your baby does not determine the relationship you will have with the baby. You do that in fun ways that we will start to really explore after we talk about the monumental task of feeding a baby.

The Golden Hour

For photographers, the golden hour is the time just after sunrise or right before sunset. The bright glare of the day hasn't begun or is over, and a soft spectrum of light touches the ground. The world is suddenly and briefly picture perfect. Hospital lighting will never be as grand as the rotating sun. However, when a newborn emerges crying at the dawn of their lives, it becomes the golden hour of yours.

The golden hour after delivery is the hour right after birth when skin to skin with the newborn and the birth parent is encouraged and hopefully supported. People think this is meant to help you bond immediately with the baby, but strong bonds take time to develop. While there is some science describing how cuddling a baby after delivery helps herald hormonal changes to promote secure attachments, there is more to the golden hour. The hours and first few days after delivery are critical for milk production in lactating parents. Remember, *transition* is a medical term describing how infants cope with their emergence into the world. Placing the newborn on your chest and letting them cuddle may assist with temperature regulation and breathing control. However, the most important benefit to having your baby on your chest is establishing an immediate breastfeeding journey with them.

The first few days after birth are critical for breastfeeding. Remember this if you, a friend, or a relative wants to try breastfeeding. Having the baby on your chest right after delivery readies the body for the process of milk production. If milk production is not supported immediately, each passing hour represents a missed opportunity for it to start. The science here is strong: the golden hour helps you make gold-colored colostrum, that first protein-rich milk that coats and fills a baby's stomach in small and vital quantities. Health care professionals should do everything they can to support the birth parent and baby to establish breastfeeding, deferring elective checks or procedures whenever possible no matter how short or long breastfeeding may be for. The importance of the golden hour is what makes some parents feel so stressed about breastfeeding early on.

The Gold Standard for Nutrition

Many formulas wish they could be breast milk. Formula companies often try to make formula as close to breast milk as they possibly can. As a result, formula is an excellent form of nutrition for infants. But when Aunt Regina tells you your cousin was only fed formula and now your cousin is a doctor, so therefore formula is just as good as breast milk, she's using her personal experiences, not scientific fact, to make conclusions. Even though her story showcases a success, her conclusions can still be wrong. Formula is great, but breast milk is better. It is the best nutrition for *most* infants. So, if you can breastfeed or offer breast milk—even for a short amount of time—you should try. Here's why.

I'll give it to formula; in certain ways it does a great job of copying breast milk. Centuries of trying to mimic breast milk led to the discovery that cow's milk was an adequate mammal mimicker of human milk (note: some cultures and formulas also use goat's milk). As a result, most formulas are sourced from cow's milk proteins. Those proteins can be modified to try to match the proteins in human milk. Fats, sugars, vitamins, and minerals are also adjusted to resemble human milk, and do a good job of it. However, human milk has a *je ne sais quoi* that formula never will; it changes. Human milk adapts to meet the needs of a growing infant. The components of formula are static and have a shelf life; they aren't capable of change—not like you, me, and breast milk are. In addition to containing different proteins and having the ability to flex, human milk has hormones. These hormones cross over from birth parent to baby. They help the baby relax, regulate their hunger, and provide stimulation for growth.

In addition, breast milk has tremendous anti-inflammatory, antimicrobial, and immune-boosting benefits. If you want to give your baby a healthy start, human milk as nutrition does just that. It contains proteins like antibodies that can fight infection and living immune cells to help shield infants from bacteria and viruses. This doesn't mean your baby will never get ill, but they will be better protected than a formula-fed baby, especially in the first year after birth. Breast milk is not only the most comprehensive nutrition, it's real medicine. This means less time at the doctor's office, fewer antibiotics, and some peace of mind for parents. If more birth parents breastfed, it would mean fewer sick babies hanging out in the hospital. This is how and why breast milk gets pushed as a public health initiative; it's a strategy to protect your community.

Alright, Well, if I Can't Use My Milk, I'll Use Other Humans'!

Donor breast milk is a term we throw around a lot in the neonatal intensive care unit (NICU) because we prefer human milk to any form of cow's milk for our preterm babies. Human milk means better growth and less infection in babies born early with weaker immune systems; however, even parents of full-term babies seek out human milk from neighbors, friends, and online groups when they want to use it, or when breastfeeding just isn't going well for them. There is a difference between milk donated to a human milk bank and milk donated to you directly from another person, so let's talk about it.

If you get milk from a friend it keeps some of its nutrients, but it's better to get milk from a bank, as you know it's pasteurized and checked for any concerns for infection. If you obtain milk from a human milk bank, you are getting milk donated by other lactating parents. Maybe they had an oversupply, or they cut their breastfeeding journey short and had milk left over, or maybe they suffered the loss of a baby and wanted to donate milk in remembrance of them. There are so many reasons parents give this amazing gift. For more information on donating human milk please use this QR code.

Donated human milk is first screened. You can think of the screening for donor milk as similar to the screening when donating blood. Medical and lifestyle questions are asked to see if you are an eligible donor. These screeners tend to be conservative and want lactating individuals to be off medications if possible. Next, they will ask about testing for various infections, such as HIV (human immunodeficiency virus), which can pass in breast milk to the infant. So, families donating through a milk bank have to be ok with sharing their medical records from the obstetrician. Lastly, the donating parent signs a contract and is educated on pumping, storage, and hygiene moving forward. When the milk is received by the bank, it's pasteurized. Yup, pasteurized just like the milk you buy in the store. This pasteurization process removes any harmful viruses or bacteria. It also changes the nutritional components of proteins in the milk, and any processing of milk removes some calories from fat. So it's kind of like a "skim" milk. It's not just the fat that's skimmed from the milk; it's important to mention the immune properties that make breast milk good at protecting from infection—things like antibodies—are all deactivated with the pasteurization process. So while the digestability and nutritional content is similar, the immune benefits just aren't there with donor milk.

A potential downside to this milk is that it's expensive, more so than formula. Formula costs about $1 a day for a baby, whereas donor milk is about $9 per day. You can buy donor milk from a lot of milk banks without any medical justification. However, in some cases, families can get the cost of donor milk covered by their insurance and there is a lot of good advocacy in this area trying to get coverage for more families. As you can imagine, though, anything dealing with insurance coverge is not easy and takes some paperwork and doctors' notes. Check your state laws on this because some states (yay Pennsylvania!) are supportive of donor milk usage…and some are less so.

Donated milk does have some advantages over formula. You can use it for up to 4 hours after defrosting, whereas formula has to be used within an hour after preparation. Additionally, you can refrigerate donor milk for up to 72 hours to keep it fresh (we will talk a little bit more about human milk storage in a minute), and premade formula has to be used within 24 hours. Formula is more readily available, though, while donor milk is a more limited resource. So, often donor milk is reserved for infants who need it the most—like our preterm infants in the NICU.

Baby Friendly, Birth Parent Frosty

When we talk about relationship building with an infant, birth parents may think breastfeeding is critical to this. Many know breast milk is good for babies, and they think breastfeeding is when true connections are built. Breastfeeding meshes with bonding, with feelings of self-worth, and it collides with a birth parent's mental health. This impact can translate into magical fireworks, or a terrible clash of glorious expectations with a difficult reality. Breastfeeding and birth parent mental health are intertwined. If your doctors aren't addressing both simultaneously, you aren't getting the support you need.

Many birth parents may recall a pressure to breastfeed right at birth, in that golden hour we talked about. To a certain extent this is true because of how beneficial it is to establish your milk supply. I have walked into rooms to double-check on families that want to use formula in the hospital. I want to provide any helpful information or answer any questions they might have to support breastfeeding. This is because the first minutes, hours, and weeks after your baby is born are critical for preparing the body to make milk. Without consistent support and stimulation at the breast, a person's full milk supply may not come in. Any desire to provide breast milk or feed at the chest could be lost. I don't want to make decisions for families, but I want them to understand how their decisions could affect their milk supply. I find that important. What's one of the main reasons birth parents who start breastfeeding stop? It's because they perceive they have an insufficient or low milk supply in the first 1 to 4 weeks after delivery. Few things truly meet the basic economic principle of supply and demand, but breastfeeding and the production of human milk do. There is a real urgency to discuss breastfeeding right away and help support breastfeeding from the moment a baby is born. Along with, you know, the immense pressures of taking care of a new human and building a relationship with them. It's a lot.

Neonatologists and pediatricians feel this breastfeeding urgency, and in their own ways try to make sure families know about breastfeeding. We start discussing and promoting breastfeeding right after birth. I ask parents if they want information; again, I am trying to

help, not hurt. All hospital staff, including nurses and lactation con-
sultants, are taught to do the same. Remember, I mentioned breastfeeding as a public health initiative, and this one has gone global:
enter the Baby-Friendly Hospital Initiative (BFHI). The BFHI started
in 1991 as a collaboration between the World Health Organization
(WHO) and the United Nations Children's Fund (UNICEF), and it
was meant to give parents the encouragement and tools they needed
to breastfeed. So here in the United States, we took this planet-wide
program and tried to structure it to work within our hospitals. The
problem with public health initiatives of this scale is they tend to
support a "one size fits all" mentality and try spreading information to large groups of diverse people without recognizing them as
individuals. Birth parents in Estonia are receiving the same basic
information as birth parents in Brazil. However, even when equipped
with the same information, they may act and feel very differently
about breastfeeding based on the culture in which they live, their
social supports, and their individual goals.

What BFHI has done is expose a gaping void in America: the
lack of community and federal support for lactating individuals. The
rollout of baby-friendly hospital environments to promote breastfeeding right after birth came without appropriate recognition of
the resources, time, and support a parent needs to breastfeed *after*
leaving the hospital. Yes, step 10 does say, "Foster the establish-
ment of breastfeeding support groups and refer mothers to them
on discharge from the hospital or clinic"—but to what extent every
community can do this looks different. Additionally, BFHI doesn't
address the mental health of the parents attempting to accomplish a
very personal and physically demanding task. It just puts everything
on the rounded shoulders of a lactating individual hunched over
their baby. Breastfeeding your baby without time and support—you
can do it! It can be hard to do it, and many families have challenges.
While education on the time-sensitive nature of breastfeeding and

help with latching the baby on day 1 (or day zero) is great, forming peer support groups and finding lactation support on day 3 when you are at home is really difficult. The Centers for Disease Control and Prevention (CDC) highlights that without maternity leave, affordable child care, or laws to protect a birth parent's ability to pump and provide for their children, the best-laid plans to try to breastfeed cannot be milked for all they're worth. In the United States, we acknowledge that breast milk is the best nutrition for infants, but we do little to support and sustain breastfeeding in our communities. Looking at the CDC data, around 83% of families try breastfeeding, around half are doing it at 6 months, and only 35% or so are continuing at 1 year. In 2022, the American Academy of Pediatrics recommended that families breastfeed as a sole source of nutrition for 6 months and for up to 2 years or longer as desired. Exhausted parents are wondering what is going wrong, whom can they turn to, and why they feel so blue.

Postpartum Blues and Depression Cues

If you are feeling sad and overwhelmed with feeding a new baby, you are not alone. Postpartum depression and related mood and anxiety disorders are common. So prevalent, in fact, you can pretty much expect to have the blues; up to 80% of new birth parents do in some form. Ultimately, though, it is not your job to assess your mental health while simultaneously recovering and caring for someone else. Wherever you deliver, make sure a health care professional screens you for postpartum mood and anxiety disorders, or worse, postpartum psychosis. Generally, the screens are a series of questions about your mood and are known to recognize if the feelings you are having are typical or require more support. Anxiety is sometimes the entryway to depression, so feeling anxious can lead to depression if you aren't watching how you worry.

Am I making you anxious? Let's do a thought exercise together. Reflect on the time you ran to catch a train or a bus, or maybe you were just walking down the street and stepped off a curb and, boom, you injured your foot or leg. My husband has broken his fifth metatarsal, a tiny bone in the foot going out to the pinkie toe, a total of 3 times by rolling his foot in fun directions while just trying to walk. If accidents like this don't happen to you, just think about a time your body told you it needed a break. Each time my husband broke a bone, he was in pain, which is no fun. In addition, he was depressed about having to use crutches or wear a boot to get around. His quality of life changed. Setting aside a busy schedule to slow down and let it heal was frustrating, and needing support to do things he previously could was humbling and made him sad.

Now, consider the birth parent's position. For around 10 months, a human being was growing inside their body. They might feel deconditioned and unable to do the same exercises and movements they did before the baby. During pregnancy, people commented on the birth parent's body, how it was changing, what they looked like ("Your belly is so cute!"). There is no escape from the changes. Next comes the physical act of pushing this person out of their body or undergoing an abdominal surgery for the baby to be born. If you imagined how depressing it might be to have an ankle sprain or a busted toe, think about trying to use the bathroom when your undercarriage lacks muscular reinforcement. I'll tell you from experience, it really stings. On top of the physical pain, a postpartum body can be unrecognizable to the parent. A now empty uterus can leave birth parents feeling depleted and physically deflated—stretch marks, saggy skin, and all. A popped balloon that's lost its air. So here you are, recovering from something both excruciating and exhilarating, and you have no time to devote to it because there is this new person you just gave birth to. On top of that, somehow there is a societal expectation that you will get your old body back. After everything you went through, once you give birth to the baby, you can somehow be your old self again. Herein lies the tension: basking in the true miracle of life on the one hand and experiencing the pain and sacrifice of having your body change and adapt on the other hand. Also, if someone hasn't been through child-birth, they don't understand you will never be the same again. Because after demanding so much of yourself throughout pregnancy, birth is only the beginning of changing demands on your time and energy. Breastfeeding is one of those demands, and it's a significant one.

After giving birth, you are being asked to form a relationship with a new person while your relationship with yourself is in flux. Most birth parents have a physical check-in with their doctors any-where from 4 to 6 weeks after they deliver. This is too long to wait to have a mental health check-in with yourself because how you are feeling will influence how you will interact with your newborn. Try not to do this alone. Having people around to support you is import-ant; these people are integral to your and your baby's health. If you are spending 24/7 with your infant and not taking time to recover, this is not going to make you a better parent and it's not going to strengthen your relationship with your baby. It might hurt it.

What does this have to do with breastfeeding? In a word, every-thing. Many who breastfeed think it's all on them. They have the breasts and the milk and are the only people who can feed their baby. That is an immense amount of pressure on a person who just gave birth and who must figure out a new relationship with themselves and their infant. Breastfeeding is a group project; one person cannot do all the work. When you have breastfeeding advocates and sup-port around you, you will experience more success at breastfeeding your baby, and often you will do it for longer. Support people aren't just partners, husbands, or fathers. They are grandparents, aunts, uncles, doulas, night nurses, siblings, and anyone who is going to be there for you after you deliver. Talk to the people who will love and nourish you after delivery and discuss the ways in which you want to nourish your baby. Get on the same page about how you want to feed the baby because you will be doing a lot of feeding after the baby is born.

Health care professionals always talk about what you want to feed your baby, and those conversations generally include questions like the following:

- What type of milk do you want to use? Breast milk? Donated human milk? Formula? Alternating or mixing feeds (realizing that if you want to use breast milk, you need to invest in your supply early on)?
- How do you want to feed the baby? At the breast? With a bottle? With both?
- Who will be feeding the baby?
- Will you be pumping? Do you have supplies for that?
- If you are buying formula, where will you be getting it? Do you have any ready for delivery?

If you are thinking you want to do any breastfeeding, it's good to educate yourself about common pitfalls (we will review some in a minute). That way, when you come up against them, especially early on while you are recovering, you will be more prepared to tackle them. Knowing that they are common may help you continue with breastfeeding if that is your goal. Stopping is always an option if your emotional health and well-being are truly suffering, but everyone experiences some issues when they are starting out and learning how to feed an infant at the breast. Even if it's your fifth baby, you don't know how the relationship is going to work until you try it.

Let me stress again, breastfeeding is not just between the birth parent and baby. Identify support people. This is important for your mental health, but it is also important for your success at breastfeeding. It might feel like since you are the only person breastfeeding you must do it by yourself. Remember you cannot. Breastfeeding is a team sport. There are many things a support person can do. They can start by being on the same page as you about how you want your baby to feed—at the breast, with a bottle, with breast milk, with some formula, or with only formula. Discuss your milk preferences for your baby before they are born. Next, work to educate yourself and anyone caring for a baby about what it takes to breastfeed, so when challenges occur, everyone will be on the same page about what can be done. It is normal to feel overwhelmed and sad in the first 2 weeks after delivery; see if you can navigate the common challenges. Following are questions and comments I get from a lot of parents just starting out with breastfeeding. Tackle these items as a team, so you can make the most of your breastfeeding journey for your family.

Questions and Comments I Often Get From My Patients

I'm not making enough milk. What can I do?

You are…and you aren't. The first milk that is produced is something called colostrum. It occurs in very low quantities but is protein rich. You would feel much fuller eating a half-pound of chicken than you would scarfing down the same weight in cookies. To be clear, I'm all about eating cookies when you are breastfeeding. The point I'm trying to make is that protein-rich foods, and colostrum is protein rich, make you feel fuller in smaller quantities. Thus, even though your baby is taking in small volumes of milk in the beginning, it should be filling for them. You aren't expected to produce a robust or mature milk supply until about day 3 to 5 of breastfeeding.

Whether or not your baby requires additional milk to help them is separate from exactly how much milk you are producing if breastfeeding. I did not get honors (which is the equivalent of an A+) in my pediatrics rotation in medical school because I forgot to ask families a very important question. During my rotation I was supposed to ask families how they know an infant is feeding well, and that answer was supposed to include how many wet or dirty diapers the baby puts out. This is good to know because it's a good marker of the infant's hydration status. In addition to their urine and stool output, monitoring their weight and jaundice levels is key to making sure they are getting good hydration. Try to focus less on how much milk you are producing and more on signs the infant is getting enough milk to be hydrated, particularly in those early days of breastfeeding.

What should I do when my baby is just so sleepy, they don't want to breastfeed?

Your baby, like you, is recovering from the delivery. It is common for babies to be sleepy, and for you to be tired too. Not all babies are like this, mind you—some are awake and ready to go. (For more information on crying see Chapter 8.) In general babies sleep up to 18 hours a day in fun and unpredictable spurts. In practice, though, it's a drag, one of the hardest things about having a newborn. It's not that your day zero (or 1) baby isn't interested in eating; most babies wake up on day 2 (or 1) and are ravenous. Until the baby is ready to tell you about feeds, you should just keep trying to get them to the breast or on a bottle 8 to 12 times in a 24-hour period (don't go more than 4 hours between feeds or you won't squeeze these sessions in), and that the infant is actively feeding for at least 10 minutes when they make an attempt at feeding. The more they do skin to skin with you and stimulate your nipples, the more they will coax your milk supply to come in. Some people lean on the folk knowledge that you shouldn't wake a sleeping baby, but in the first few weeks after birth, that adage doesn't apply. While newborns have some fat, they don't have enough to keep their sugar levels up. Adults also store some sugar in their liver, but a baby's liver is immature. I say sugar because milk contains lactose, which is a sugar. That lactose breaks down into other simpler sugars that the developing brain needs to fuel itself. So, skipping feeds might drop sugar levels and make focusing on feeds essential in these sleepy newborns. Any guess what? If you skip a feed and your sugar levels are low that makes you more sleepy—so you cannot skip feeds. Babies born preterm or premature (less than 37 weeks' gestation) or early term (in the 37-week zone) tend to be the biggest sleepyheads. So don't let them snooze; feeding is now your full-time job.

So how do you wake a sleeping baby? There is a reason for the phrase "sleeping like a baby." Sometimes, loud noises or bright lights won't do the trick. To wake babies, I like to take off their clothes, change their diapers, and keep them naked at the breast so we can truly be skin to skin. It's always stimulating to be naked. Then sometimes I'll lightly tap their feet or blow in their face—if I'm not feeling sick—to tickle them. In the delivery room you might notice the pediatric specialists stroking the baby's spine to make them cry. That's a great tactic for getting them to open up their lungs and transition from the watery womb to breathing air. It's not a great way to wake them for breastfeeding, as they will arch and not latch well. So if you are going to tickle their bodies do it down their sides so they wiggle and curl up into you. These tactics often rouse sleepy babies to attempt feeds. Don't wait for the baby to cry to tell you they are hungry; if they are awake and rooting around, they probably are interested in feeding. While rooting around is a fun term to throw around, it's also a reflex in babies. A hungry baby will suck on any-thing that gets close to their mouth—a hand, a shirt, a nose—that's a signal they are ready to feed! Really hungry babies will put their hands up to their mouths and you made need someone to help hold their hands down so they can latch onto the breast well. So it's always good to get some help getting baby on the breast as you figure out their movements and cues.

The baby is feeding nonstop! Why does it feel like they are so greedy?

Breastfeeding a newborn is a full-time job. It gets easier with time and practice, but in the beginning, clear your schedule and pencil in feedings around the clock. This is your new profession. You won't have time for anything else. This might not be ok for you…and that's ok. It can be hard to breastfeed constantly—that's why it's a family affair or a group effort. For you to breastfeed, the other things or people you are responsible for need attention, and a good support person can provide that. It also might be comforting to know there is wisdom to babies' spending a lot of time at the breast in the beginning. It's like they know the more time they spend at the breast, the faster your milk might come in. So that's where they want to be. This phenomenon is often called cluster feeding, but from the parent's perspective it should be called "What am I doing wrong?" feeding or "I can't keep this this up" feeding. Lactating individuals perceive that the baby is fussy and unsatisfied, and perceive themselves as already having failed at breastfeeding and the entire relationship they are trying to build with their little loved one as not going well. Cluster feeding, though, is short lived once your milk supply gets revved up. So there is hope. Breastfeeding is a journey, and the destination is dependent on what you desires and goals are for feeding.

When a baby is really wanting the breast or to eat—that's when greedy baby remarks start to happen. To me, greed has negative connotations. Through the years I've learned that for some parents it's a term of frustration, but it also can be a term of pride or endearment. "My baby is so greedy, and they feed so well!" Greed is defined as an intense or selfish desire for something. As such, I think for the baby it's a complex emotion they can't really feel. Yes, they want to eat a ton in the first few days after birth, particularly after the first 24 hours. However, it's unclear if they are capable of being selfish. It's

not that they lack consideration for others; they are just functioning at
a biological and primal level to survive. Again, it's as if they know the
more time they spend at the breast, the faster your body can make the
milk. To me, it's not greedy, it's actually pretty smart as an adaptation
for survival. I prefer to call my cluster feeders smart, not greedy.

I am sore; will this stop hurting?

Your nipples might hurt from breastfeeding in the beginning.
Nipples are so sensitive, and having someone suck on them isn't an
everyday occurrence for most. When someone tells me it hurts when
they breastfeed, I need more information. I often want to look at
the nipples—and a good pediatrician should be able to do a quick
assessment of the nipples to help with referrals for feeding issues.
Are they cracked? Creased? Lipstick shaped? Bleeding? Inverted, or
not popping out? If the nipples are intact and their shape is typical,
I'll provide reassurance. If they look torn up or aren't rounded and
erect, I'll often want to assess the infant's latch or ask an experienced
lactation consultant to help me do that. Because an improper latch
at the breast can be the reason why there is pain. You want to get to
the bottom of this right away because an improper latch also means
there is likely not as much milk expression occurring to prime your
body for milk production. Remember, the first few days after a baby
is born represent a critical window for supply. Plus, there are things
a lactation specialist can do to address a faulty latch. They can assess
the baby by looking at the roof of the mouth and the movement of
their facial muscles and tongue. For sore nipples I also really recommend nipple creams (like lanolin) or butters (usually with natural
bases like olive oil) from the get-go to keep the nipple in good shape.
Birth parents may also find their own breast milk on the nipple
has healing qualities. Cold gels represent yet another really helpful
source for sore nipples—so there are things you can find to help! If

the nipples are inverted, it can sometimes hurt to have them pop out, and in the short term a lactation expert might recommend something called a nipple shield. It used to shield a nipple to either protect it or elongate it so a baby has a way to latch on well.

Pain can also arise from the breast itself. Usually, breast pain does not occur in the hospital, but you may feel it around days 3 to 5 when the breasts become filled with milk. If you remember my story of a clogged milk duct, full breasts can get hot, stretchy, and painful. This is called engorgement and represents a blossoming milk supply. So exciting your milk is in, not so exciting your breasts feel like swollen, oversized cantaloupes. At this point, they also might leak milk unexpectedly—so back to nipples. You can get nipple pads to soak up leaky milk or milk catchers to put over your nipples to try to save the milk for later.

Does my baby have a tongue-tie?

If you have been reading this book closely you probably thought I was delinquent in the physical exam section. In examining the mouth, I never mention looking for a tongue-tie. Why? Because tongue-ties or ankyloglossia cannot be diagnosed with one physical exam move. We all have a piece of tissue that connects our tongue to the base of our mouth. Sometimes that tissue can "tie up" the tongue and make it hard for the tongue to move and create a good suck for baby. Sometimes when the baby moves the tongue they can't stick it all the way out of the mouth. These are all clues tongue movement for sucking might be impaired—but no 2 babies are alike. And one baby might have these exam findings and eat just fine, while another might have them and eat poorly. During the first few days after birth for a baby there are so so so many things that affect feeds and even if there might be a tongue-tie (again, there is not one physical exam maneuver to diagnose it) that might not be the reason a baby will feed poorly.

The diagnosis and treatment of tongue-tie has skyrocketed recently. The treatment includes a procedure either with scissors or with a laser to release the tissue underneath the tongue. The procedure is often well tolerated by the baby especially soon after birth; however, there can be complications, particularly with the laser procedure, from which there can be scarring and burns that might make the baby's feeding issues worse. So if someone recommends this procedure to you here are a few things you MUST do before getting it.

1. Get a second opinion—from a pediatrician, lactation consultant, speech therapist trained with infants (emphasis on the training), or an occupational therapist also with infant training.
2. Ask if there are other ways to address the potential tongue-tie with exercises, different feeding positions, or special baby sucking/chew toys.
3. Make sure the procedure is covered by your insurance when you get this diagnosis. A big fear of many pediatricians is diagnosis and treatment of tongue-tie has been profit driven and preyed on parental anxiety about feeds—so give yourself time and be thoughtful about who is giving your baby this release.

To illustrate how difficult it is to diagnose a tongue-tie—my third baby's tongue-tie wasn't diagnosed until 4 months after birth. Generally, infants with a significant tongue-tie will feed poorly; for my baby, it was the 4-month weight check that let on that there was an issue. Some other symptoms of a tongue-tie could be pain with breastfeeding, seeing a tight or thick piece of tissue under the tongue, the inability to stick the tongue out over the gums. Or a heart-shaped appearance of the tongue, a clicking sound with feeds, and an inability for the baby to stay latched for long. In retrospect, my baby always clicked their tongue with feeds and popped on and off the breast frequently. That said, I never had any pain with feeds and had such a strong milk letdown from being a third-time breastfeeding parent (good news—you usually make more milk with each baby, yay) I didn't notice a change in diaper frequency and baby always seems happy and satiated after their small feeds. This diagnosis came as a blow to me because my other babies didn't have feeding issues and I tried to do everything right. I got lactation support early on, I monitored my infant's hydration status; I was pretty shook up about the weight and I took it personally.

Ultimately, no one in my care team could strongly recommend a tongue-tie release. I chatted with my pediatrician, got my lactation consultant back, and got the help of a trusted pediatric speech therapist in my community. There was not going to be a clear benefit for my baby in its release. Because my decision was to continue breastfeeding, as baby seemed to be developing normally despite her small size, my plan moving forward was more frequent smaller volume feeds, fortification of feeds with some formula (starting at around 6 to 7 months), special bottle nipples that were long and allowed for her to get her tongue around them better, and stretching exercises for the tongue. I found toys that were long and narrow for her to practice her suck or that allowed her to stick her tongue out (think a honeycomb ball you often see babies play with), and more weight checks-in with my pediatrician. If it was guaranteed a tongue-tie release would have solved her feeding issues, absolutely I would have done it. But, having a slightly older baby who was otherwise content—I was content with extra monitoring and exercises as opposed to an intervention that might cause her pain without any benefit to her feeds.

There is often no quick fix to feeding issues. Some babies—tongue-tie or not—are going to have a sucky suck and need supports to feed. This is why building a trusted support team and recognizing what your goals are and how flexible you can be with them are so important when feeding a baby. I had pressure to just stop breastfeeding and monitor everything my baby ate with a bottle. But at the end of the day—it wasn't like the bottle was easier for her to suck on, and we enjoyed our feeds together. So, I pumped more to maintain a supply and I kept breastfeeding her with the more frequent feeds mentioned previously. I don't regret it, not one bit. This was the last baby I was going to feed. But I recognize it was extra time and mental energy I was using to keep breastfeeding going and that was hard on me. But it was my decision to keep going, because breastfeeding meant a lot to both of us. I will always think it was worth it for those 10 minutes at night when I breastfed her to bed in a quiet room and we cuddled and I couldn't imagine being anywhere else in the world.

I am feeling overwhelmed. Can I feed formula?

How you feed your baby is your decision. Not your grandmothers', your doctors', your nurses', your sisters', your cousins', your neighbors'— your choice. Consider the opinion of your most trusted partner for caring for baby, as they should be tracking your mental health and stamina to breastfeed. If your baby is being fed consistently and with care, it can be done in any number of ways. Mixed feeding is when use of breast milk is supplemented with use of some formula— maybe right from the beginning. The use of any breast milk is simply amazing because breast milk is almost always the most sophisticated and nutrient-rich milk out there. This is what you need to remember: The amount of time you breastfeed and the time the baby spends at the breast in the first few days after delivery are going to have a huge impact on your supply later. The early moments count. They matter a lot. When you offer formula over breastfeeding and don't stimulate the body to let it know it needs to produce (aka pump when offering a formula bottle), you are setting yourself up to make less milk.

Some parents tell me they want to rely on mixed feedings until their milk comes in because they are worried the baby will be hungry. I explain to them that it's typical for their body to not make a lot of milk in the beginning, that there are ways to make sure the baby is satiated.

If breastfeeding is the desired feeding method, then I stress focusing on it instead of worrying about supplementation right off the bat. To wait and see what happens to the baby's weight, diaper counts, and physical exam to look for hydration over the first 2 to 3 days. For some families, I even recommend pumping to stimulate the milk supply and supplementation with breast milk if I'm worried about them not having a good supply right away—say the baby was born slightly premature and has a weaker latch, or they had a breast reduction and we aren't sure how much breast tissue they have to make milk.

Remember, some infants won't take to the breast even with support, and that's ok. Parenthood quickly teaches you that it's hard to get everything you want from your relationship with your baby. When you are using your body to feed, decide how much of it you want to give and how far you are willing to push yourself to meet your goals. Realize that you might not be able to have everything the way you planned.

I just want to pump; none of this baby on the breast.

Breasts are sexualized in American society. Having someone at the breast, even if it's your child, can feel upsetting for some people. They might not want to directly breastfeed because it doesn't feel right or it's emotionally triggering.

It's not just the physical act of breastfeeding that can feel off. Anticipating the need to feed when out with an infant also can make mothers uncomfortable. Some struggle with breastfeeding in public places, and it gives them pause or anxiety. You have the right to feed your baby anywhere. So don't let puritanical notions dictate if you can directly breastfeed your baby. Again, that's a decision you make about your body. There are a growing number of public spaces for mothers to pump and breastfeed their infants. I breastfed anywhere I wanted to and wasn't shy about the mammalian use of my breasts. They are not just ornamental after all.

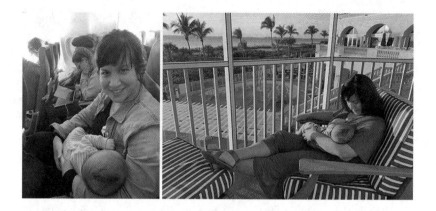

Pumping You Up to Pump

There is a subset of birth parents who cannot directly breastfeed their infants. Maybe it has something to do with the nipple or the breast shape or anatomy. It might be that the infant doesn't have the appropriate latch because of the shape of their mouth or their muscular control. Many times, there are workarounds for these issues, so that is why early lactation support is critical. But at times, getting the baby to the breast just isn't really an option.

If the baby can't get milk out of the breast, a pump often can. We often don't recommend pumping early on as we want the baby to set the pace and establish the milk supply. For those who want to directly breastfeed, hand expression during a baby's first days often is a more successful way to stimulate and care for the breast, as well as to get milk. It takes some practice and, admittedly, I was never very good at it, so I enjoyed a mechanical pump more than my own 2 hands.

Pump technology has finally been catching up to the needs of mothers. Insurance coverage is getting there but is less than all-encompassing. So always check with your insurance about what pumps are covered for you when choosing. It's nice to have a pump that is portable. Some need to be plugged in to function, which can be cumbersome. Others are bulky, so not great on the move. Think about the weight, size, and ability to carry the pump if you are thinking it will travel with you when the baby can't. Now there are pumps that fit into your bra, making pumping on the go that much easier. Your breasts generally do get bigger with lactation, and the pump inside your undergarments makes your cup size go up considerably. I had one, and no one seemed to notice as much as I did.

It's also helpful to use a more common brand of pump. Pump parts can get lost or break, so having a brand name product will make it easier for you to find replacement parts when you need them. If pumping is part of the feeding plan, bring your pump to the hospital when you deliver. That way you can learn how to use it with a lactation consultant (they are generally with you postpartum, as most birth hospitals will have them). A major thing to know is your flange size—the pump part that goes around the nipple. You want a comfortable fit on your areola, but the nipple itself needs to move freely under the plastic. I didn't figure out how to use my pump until the first day back at work. I don't recommend using that very stressful approach. Finding a good fit and knowing the mechanics of the pump early on could save you from emotional moments on the go.

For those reading this, if you can come up with a way to clean pump parts efficiently and nightly, let's talk. I'll quit my job as a neonatologist and join your startup for clean pump parts. Cleaning pump parts can be tedious and time consuming. As someone who had to pump almost every day at work, I was cleaning my pump parts every night. The sanitation process involves use of boiling or steaming water, followed by daily washing with soap and water along with air-drying. I was hesitant to use the dishwasher because my pump parts were plastic and I didn't want them to become warped or to have chemicals leach from the plastic. Saving pumped milk also requires dexterity with packaging, pouring, and storing.

So the pumping process needs to be factored into your day and night with your baby, or delegated to one of your support people. Some people pump exclusively and they are heroes of the breast milk world. Check in on them, make sure they are feeling ok, and marvel at their grit and dedication to making milk.

Milk Storage: Saving the Pumped Parts

After you pump milk, you must put it somewhere. I didn't reach my breastfeeding goals with my first baby, so fueled by determination, grit, and arguably some degree of postpartum insanity I began storing milk right away with my second. Wanting to build a vast freezer supply that I could use to reach my goals for my second breastfeeding journey.

You get to know your body when you breastfeed, and I always let milk down on both sides. With baby number 1, that meant I had to use a towel to catch the milk on the opposite side from the baby. It took me several months to find out you can buy devices to catch that milk. Some are passive and don't use any suction so are truly just bags that you attach to make sure you don't lose a drop. The one I settled on was sort of a bulky suction cup that stuck to the opposite breast and caught milk. I settled on that suction cup milk saver to make sure I was catching all the milk drops. I started using this clunky system immediately with my second, and I recommended this to many mothers. What I found was only about half of the moms who used this milk collection method were down with managing a baby and a suctioned-on silicone cup on their breasts simultaneously. I found it relatively easy with a newborn who wasn't super awake and difficult with a several-month-old baby bent on kicking it off. That's why some like the milk cups rather than the big suction cups: a little sleeker with less fuss.

Once you collect the milk, it needs to be stored. The CDC has guidelines on how to keep your milk from spoiling. For more information use this QR code.

The recommendations are nuanced, but a good rule of thumb is the rule of 4s. You can leave freshly expressed milk out on a counter for 4 hours; you can refrigerate it for up to 4 days; and you can freeze it for up to 4 months. One caveat is that you probably can freeze it for up to 6 months in a deep freezer. I bought a small secondhand *chest* freezer (no pun intended) and used it to store all of my breast milk. I also made sure to have a freezer alarm so in the off chance the power went out or the freezer became unplugged and my stash was in jeopardy, I would know. Remember, I became very dedicated to storing. Mentally, I needed that full freezer when I returned to work to feel like I had made enough milk to support my baby when I wasn't there. One postpartum thought I had as I lovingly saved my milk was that if I died, at least the baby would still have a little piece of me moving forward. I never had a plan to hurt myself or others, but my dogged mindset about breast milk probably was not the healthiest. I managed with good support structures and people around me, but professional help to allay fears of death and dying likely would have been helpful given the immense anxiety I had (and still do) about using breast milk. Hence, I firmly believe you cannot separate a birth parent's mental health from their feeding preferences. My preferences silently consumed me as I stuffed milk into the dark corners of my basement chest freezer for my third baby.

At the end of the day ample storage provided me with peace of mind, and I was lucky I could do it at all. I would say you shouldn't need to stash so much milk before you go to work if you can pump what your baby needs to eat every day you are away. But I didn't have that luxury. For all my babies, a return to work meant a dip in supply. I don't know if it was the separation or the stress of working with sick babies (it was probably both), but my breast milk supply dwindled. So I was thankful for the freezer stash and being so cognizant of pumping and storing early on.

I think this whole thing really sucks; do I have to do this?

No. You don't have to breastfeed. Although it is the gold standard of nutrition for an infant, you can choose not to do it. This does not make you a bad parent. Parenting is like taking an advanced mathematics course. Sometimes you'll logically get the answer that works, other times you will fiddle with the numbers and be unclear as to what the true answer is. While there might be times when you don't follow the best evidence-based scientific recommendations flawlessly, there will be other times when the best practices fall

---

TIPS FOR HAVING A BREAST MILK STASH

Use milk savers on the opposite breast early in lactation. This will help catch and store milk if letdown occurs on both sides (suction cup on breast or bag on breast).

You make the most milk in the morning. So when awake with baby for an early morning feed, pump afterwards to store that milk.

Consider investing in a deep freezer for milk storage so you can keep the milk fresh longer and it's not mixed in your normal fridge freezer.

If you get a freezer, invest in a freezer alarm should your power fail so you know how cold the milk stays.

To prevent waste consider storing 2 to 4 oz at a time.

seamlessly into the fabric of your life. Or maybe you will always walk somewhere in the middle. The bottom line is your infant will not love you any less for not breastfeeding. You can still have a close and loving relationship with them when using formula. Choosing not to breastfeed or being unable to doesn't mean you can't have an awesome connection with your newborn. You will have endless opportunities to connect and "brain build" that don't require breasts.

For some birth parents, the act of breastfeeding itself is depressing. An under-researched phenomenon called dysphoric milk ejection reflex (D-MER) occurs when lactating individuals feel depressed when they express milk. It's a quick and unexpected low feeling that doesn't pop up between breastfeeding or pumping sessions. These birth parents won't want to breastfeed because for them it feels unpleasant and they don't like it. Some will choose not to because they must go back to work in a few short weeks and the legal protection in place to help them pump at work aren't something they feel comfortable asking for. And some will find that bottle-feeding works better for their sanity and their baby.

What I Wish I Really Knew About Breastfeeding

In the United States in particular, the breastfeeding experiences of parents are not valued and supported. Without community resources and widespread support dedicated to breastfeeding, all the responsibility falls solely on the individual birth parent. The beginning of a breastfeeding journey can be rocky, even if there are no complications. This is because you are learning a new skill (you weren't born just knowing how to ride a bike), and this new skill requires a baby who has the reflexes and muscle control to be able to participate in it with you (you can't tango alone). Postpartum mood disorders are also prevalent and baby blues or mommy guilt can be felt in every corner of the world, and it's not always diagnosed. Birth parents are often isolated, avoiding crowds and public places to protect the health of their newborn; but at the same time, they lack the emotional and physical support that is so critical at this time and need family and friends to check in on them. The need to heal their body and build a bonding relationship with their new baby should take priority over a detailed and laborious feeding plan. The demands of breastfeeding should not be entirely on the shoulders of the individuals doing it. There should be supportive caregivers, family, and friends ready and able to provide help.

Seriously, though, this can't all fall on the shoulders of birth parents and their networks. Federal and/or state laws are needed to enhance paid parental leave everywhere. In the United States currently the only federal law protecting parental leave for families is the Family Medical Leave Act or FMLA. The catch is it's unpaid leave, you need to be in a company with more than 50 workers, and you need to have held the job for over a year. Think about that— statistically speaking only 60% of American workers qualify for FMLA; that means the other 40% don't and that's a lot of people— are you one of them? I was pregnant with my first daughter when I entered a new job and could not access the protections of FMLA. I had to rely on the generosity of my employer. That's an awkward situation to navigate when you are new on the job and experiencing your pregnancy. New families should not have to stress about having time to get to know their baby and to feed their baby right after birth—but they are here in America. We are the ONLY developed nation that cannot guarantee paid leave for families—and that is not ok. And the concept of paid leave is then left to be interpreted by individual states. There are currently 13 states (plus the District of Columbia!) that offer any form of paid leave. So check if you live in one because you are going to be able to baby bond better…and hopefully more states are added to this list by the time the book publishes. So if you are passionate about breastfeeding and about the health of children in this country, you should also be advocating and voting to protect and pay for a family leave.

I personally wish that when I had my first child, I knew the odds were stacked against me because of things out of my control (like government policies; now, though, voting for health is a pastime of mine) and that breastfeeding wasn't all on me. I wish I knew that I didn't have to carry the weight of this heavy responsibility all alone—and that there were things outside my control that made it all the more stressful. I wish when I began breastfeeding and had my own challenges and heartbreak, that there were systems around me to help me overcome and normalize them. There are some, though they can be better and tend to be community based. So, you have to start by asking your obstetrician for resources, and then pressing your pediatrician for them as well. Ask for help before you need it. Know which resources you have in your neighborhood so you can leverage them when an unexpected issue arises. By creating a plan for yourself ahead of time, you will be able to identify what you need. Identify who you can reach out to for help. All the education in the world can't always prepare you for such a physical and personal act. Having a dedicated group of champions supporting and watching out for you and baby so you can heal and achieve your feeding goals is a must. It shouldn't be a luxury afforded to only those in states supporting families—it should be the standard. So again, learn to ask for help from those around you, and be prepared to ask for help to breastfeed. Whether it all goes to plan or not, it's going to play a role in your health and your mental health after delivery. And you don't want breastfeeding to inhibit bonding, you want it to be a picture-perfect golden hour of your life you remember.

My newborn has weight loss; is that bad??

When picturing a newborn, many people think of a happy, fat little creature with a gummy toothless grin. I can tell you that newborns look neither fat nor happy; they look sort of like they got squished through something—whether that be an incision in the uterus or a vaginal canal—and they are still recovering from that initial push into the world. But the stigma about babies' bodies still exists. A newborn should be fat and happy; this is perhaps the only time in one's life that increased plumpness is praised.

I think this misconception fuels a lot of anxiety in the first week or two after delivery. Because the vast majority—almost 100% of the babies I care for—will lose weight in the first 1 to 2 weeks. This is somewhat biologically ordained. They are born with a little bit more fluid and fat than they need to get over the hump of early breastfeeding.

Early breastfeeding—especially for a first-time lactating parent—is a relationship-building activity in and of itself. The breasts should initially produce a substance called colostrum. Colostrum is often more golden in color than mature breast milk. It is the golden milk, the good stuff. Despite its low volume, colostrum is protein rich but comes in tiny volumes. It isn't until around days 3 to 5 that a person's full milk supply comes in.

This is assuming you breastfeed, but even babies fed formula or donor milk shouldn't be taking large volumes of milk in the first few days after birth. Babies' stomachs are about the size of their fists, so on day 1 we say they should be taking anywhere from 10 to 15 milliliters of milk; the amount goes up as their stomachs stretch and they get used to suckling. It isn't until around the first week after birth that they can literally stomach a full 2 ounces or 60 milliliters. This is important because when families try to give bigger volumes, say 30 milliliters or more right out of the womb, newborns often get fussy and spit up, which can cause more distress for a family just wanting to make sure the baby is fed.

So just remember, your baby doesn't want whopping milk meals early on. They want skin to skin, they want to feed frequently, and they want to sleep and work out how they are going to poop and pee. All newborns want to bond with their parents and rely on them for love and support after a traumatic event for them, as well as for the birth parent.

It is not until around day 3 or 4 that milk intake starts to pick up. That is also why I expect every baby I care for to lose weight in the first week or so after delivery. It will take time to regain that weight, just as it takes time to pick up on feeds. It's important to monitor an infant's weight after delivery, and every delivery hospital will weigh your infant daily. They are looking to see how much the baby loses, not an absolute number like, oh, 4 ounces, but a percentage of their birth weight. Any infant who loses more than 10% of their birth weight should be monitored more closely, and this is a time when it might be wise for a birth parent who is exclusively breastfeeding to supplement with pumped breast milk, donor milk, or formula. Otherwise, you can watch a baby lose some weight as long as they are otherwise well.

We live in an age of data-driven parenting. I think it can be helpful to track weight with feeds, and so having a home scale is not a crazy idea but *only if you have a pediatrician, doula, lactation consultant, or other health care professional well versed in infant care to run the numbers with you.* And I would not recommend checking a baby's weight more than once a day for the sake of your sanity and because you don't need the data. I also like to know the number of feeds in 24 hours (8 to 12 is an acceptable number), as well as the number of diaper changes (by a week or 7 days after birth you want around 7 to 8 changes a day; more are ok, fewer may be worrisome). Otherwise, as your pediatrician and friendly neonatologist, I don't need many other data about your feeds. My worry is that if you start collecting more data—timing feeds to the minute, telling me the quality and texture of every stool or urine output—you are worrying too much. And data-driven parenting seems to have heightened anxiety about parenting a newborn in general.

When to Worry About Weight: A Supplemental Guide

When does a baby need to eat more? As I explained earlier, low volumes of milk in the first few days after birth and weight loss are expected. Consider it a part of the baby's learning to eat and thrive on their own without the birth parent or placenta to help. If you decide to breastfeed, you do not need to proactively supplement your milk right after birth. You can wait at least 3 days to see what happens with the latch, the milk supply, and the baby's weight and jaundice levels.

Are there times you will need to give extra milk? Absolutely! Here are some reasons you might need to provide extra milk to your newborn right away.

- They are born prematurely or considered to be a late preterm or early term infant (anywhere from 35 to 37 weeks at birth).
- They have low blood sugar levels, which need to be addressed (this is called hypoglycemia).
- They have high bilirubin levels (jaundice), because poop helps the newborn get rid of bilirubin.
- After a few days, you notice the baby isn't getting enough milk; this usually applies to breastfed infants.
  - Weight loss is 10% of birth weight.
  - They have a delay in their bowel movements or urine output and haven't had either of those in 2 days.
  - They seem dehydrated—a pediatrician can help with this— but the baby could have a sunken fontanelle on exam, high sodium levels on laboratory checks, or increasing jaundice as mentioned earlier.

The bottom line is you don't always need to provide supple-mental milk to your newborn right out of the womb. You can give yourself and the baby a few days to figure out feeding, and newborns are programmed to take time to figure out feeds.

After the first few weeks, your pediatrician will be following a growth curve for your baby. I like to take pictures of my baby's growth curves so I can follow their percentiles with the pediatrician. Your newborn's weight when they are born is their birth weight, and the percentile is a reflection of how well the placenta supported the baby. Eventually, your baby will find their own spot on the growth curve. Some babies will be at the 90th percentile, and others will be at the fifth percentile. While weight is one objective measurement to monitor growth, development is also important, which makes going to your pediatrician in the first year so important.

Chapter 7

You Are Getting Sleepy, Very Sleepy

*A*dmitting a baby to the neonatal intensive care unit (NICU) can feel like an off-Broadway production of a gut-wrenching dramedy. The stars are a helpless baby and their frazzled family under bright white hospital lights with naked emotions. The stage for these admissions is a not-so-adorable infant hospital bed laden with alarms and marked with a cartoon giraffe. This has earned these expensive beds the name "the giraffe," which is thrown about by health care professionals when this sophisticated crib presents a technical challenge. Why is the light not working on the giraffe? The heater on the giraffe seems to be off. Wait, how do I shut off this giraffe? Can someone please help me with this giraffe?

I usually meet my patients exposed on the giraffe. They are stripped down to a diaper and lying on white sheets under the harsh light. The baby is ready to be dressed in electrocardiogram (ECG or EKG) leads, which are stickers that measure their heart rate; a temperature probe, which is a shiny golden disc also taped to their body; and a pulse oximeter that resembles a flesh-colored bandage wrapped around their foot. They also are poised for head-to-toe physical examinations to get to the diagnosis, though, in truth, an explanation (or, as doctors like to say, "history") from the family often gets you to the diagnosis faster. This was true for an infant I admitted for something called a brief resolved unexplained event, or a BRUE. Not all babies with BRUEs are admitted to the hospital, but this event had been severe. Emergency medical personnel had examined the infant in the home after a 911 call and had concerns

*about the infant's color and muscle tone. The baby was noted to be blue
and the pulse oximeter measuring the oxygen content in the blood was
below 88%, when it should have been close to 100%. Since arriving at the
hospital, the infant seemed better, but the history was compelling enough
that everyone felt the NICU was the best place to monitor them.*

*The newborn was only 7 days old and medical interventions were
already underway. Infection is something every infant needs to be
assessed for when they have a scary BRUE. Blood cultures looking for
bacteria and panels to detect viruses were taken and sent off, and antibiotics and antiviral medications were already being administered. The
baby wasn't blue now. Pink and active, the baby's eyes darted around
the room. They weren't crying, but there was a clear sense of confusion.
The birth parent sat hunched in a corner, her shoulders up around her
ears and her head in her hands. Her face was obscured in the relative
darkness outside the stage of our giraffe, and her body was in a pose
suggestive of defeat. I quickly examined the infant, and finding the exam
results to be typical for a well 7-day-old, I sat down next to the mother.*

*I introduced myself and asked her to tell me what happened, what
got us here. She started at the delivery, which had gone well. Mom
and baby were discharged from the hospital in just 24 hours, a quick
turnaround leaving much of the postdelivery recovery to happen at
home. The mother had limited help. The baby's father didn't want to
be involved in their life, but she had sisters and her mother around
for support. She tried to sleep but couldn't; anxiety about caring for
the baby kept her up every night during the baby's first week. Eventually, though, sleep found her, slowing rendering her unconscious on
the couch in her living room with her newborn cradled skin to skin
on her chest. An unknown amount of time passed. When the mother
finally awoke, her baby was no longer on her chest. The baby had slid
between her body and the couch, face and nose covered, limp and
blue. The mother sprang into action, calling 911 and starting the CPR
she learned in the hospital. Pushing on her infant's chest and blowing*

in their face between tears. When the emergency medical personnel arrived, the baby was coming to. The oxygen levels were low, and the baby was whisked away in the ambulance for further evaluation.

Sometimes for a BRUE, I'll pursue an extensive workup of cardiac examinations or measurements of brain function to figure out why the event happened. In this case, what I needed to do was sit with the mother and talk about safe sleep. Not judge her for what happened, not imply it was easy, but talk about it openly.

Your newborn will not sleep through the night. They cannot and should not sleep through the night. What does sleeping through the night mean anyway? Is it a full 8 hours? Maybe 6 hours? There is no standard definition of "sleep through the night," but the truth is you will not get a good or full night's sleep when you are caring for a newborn. That's why this chapter is here, to explain this difficult and tiring reality of newborn parenting. We will talk about infant sleep and what it looks like (see "Managing Infant Sleep" table). Sadly, in the United States, new parents are not given the support they need to be awake for the demanding job of parenting their newborn. If family leave policies allowed us to get the support and rest we need, perhaps we wouldn't be so obsessed with tracking how our baby sleeps. I see it as a reflection of how society does not support us. Here we are, though, stuck exploring strategies to help you with sleep deprivation. Because you will feel the lack of sleep when you have a newborn. So what can you do about it?

Sleep Like a Baby

Sleep is important. For your mental and physical health, and for your infant's mental and physical health. Sleep for adults is very different from what it is for babies. It's this difference between the physical needs of caregivers and infants that makes the newborn period a difficult and demanding time to parent.

Managing Infant Sleep

	INFANTS	ADULTS
Hours of sleep needed	Around 14 to 18 hours	Around 6 to 8 hours
Time asleep	Short bursts—minutes or a couple of hours	Hours at a time
Presence of circadian rhythms (understanding of day/night)	None until earliest 6 months	Sleeping at night preferred
Nutritional needs	Small meals every 3 to 4 hours, no fasting overnight	Can fast overnight, have the sugar stores (liver, fat, muscle) to do it
Control over sleep	Very little; at around 6 months of age might be able to be sleep trained	Ask for help from other caregivers as able, nap as able, find a pediatrician to talk to, provide a sleep environment that is safe, work on tools to ease sleep deprivation.

The irony of infant sleep is that they do sleep a *lot*. Up to 18 hours a day. However, that sleep is not continuous but occurs in short bursts. They wake up to feed and excrete waste, and generally fall back asleep. It can be hard to track the total sleep duration of your infant in a 24-hour period because of their frequent ups and downs. Newborns aren't doing this to challenge you as a parent, though it certainly will. They do this because it's what their body needs: plenty of down time to grow and around-the-clock nourishment to keep their bodies and brains healthy and fed. There is this Western notion that infants, especially after the first few weeks following birth, should be sleeping "through the night." People have these expectations for babies without realizing they *can't* sleep through the night. These expectations get families into trouble.

Because infant sleep is not what a grown-up body needs. Adults crave uninterrupted periods of sleep, while infants need to be tended to around every 2 to 4 hours. This leads to anxiety, which pediatricians know can lead to depression and is hard on first-time parents. As someone with medical training who was asked routinely to stay up for 24 to 30 hours at a time, or to work night shifts ranging from 10 to 14 hours, I thought I would be prepared for sleep deprivation

and embrace it with my newborn. The difference is that in my medical training, a 24-hour shift was usually followed by a 24-hour period
when I could just lie on the couch and watch TV or attempt to sleep.
When a person is depending on you for survival, the time off just
never comes; you must be *on* constantly and that drives your cumu-
lative sleep hours to new lows. Parenting a newborn means being
vigilant, and sleep falls to the wayside because you want to be there
for your baby. And somehow in just 3 short months (if you are lucky)
after an almost 10-month pregnancy, you are expected to resume a
normal work schedule as if the whole baby thing is done, when really
your altered life has only just begun.

Let's go deeper into what "sleeping through the night" might
mean. When people are asked about it, generally they will say that
sleeping through the night for a newborn means anywhere from
6 to 8 hours without interruption. In a study from *Pediatrics,*
"Uninterrupted Infant Sleep, Development, and Maternal Mood,"
(2018;142[6]:e20174330. https://doi.org/10.1542/peds.2017-4330),
hundreds of parents were surveyed about their infants' sleep habits;
only about half said their infants could sleep for 6 hours at a time by
age 6 months. And only around 40% of parents said their babies could
sleep for 8 hours at a time at 6 months of age, leaving more than half
of infants unable to sleep for that long a stretch. So, for months babies
don't really have the ability to sleep for more than a few hours at a
time. This is typical and something to brace yourself for. Infants' sleep
patterns vary, but overwhelmingly they will not sleep in long stretches;
this is especially true for newborns. It's worth repeating: infant sleep is
unpredictable and your infant *will* keep you up at night. This should be
the expectation.

A friend of mine once said she lied to her pediatrician about her
infant's sleeping through the night. She didn't want the doctor to judge
her for being up with the baby, and it was easier to lie than explain how
she was dealing, both physically and emotionally, with her fractured

sleep. As a rule, be completely honest about what's going on in your home. Your pediatrician will help support you and provide suggestions or tips for either normalizing infant sleep or thinking of ways to help you and the baby sleep better if that's your goal. You cannot force your baby to sleep through the night; they are not programmed to do that. You can find a pediatrician who will support and guide you through this very tough phase of parenting. This is something you *can* control. Your relationship with your pediatrician matters because not only do you need to go to them with your infant's medical issues, but you need to fold them into your parenting journey as well. It's good to know the things you *can* control! You can control your infant's sleep environment, and you should make it safe. Then you should spend some time thinking about the parent you want to be, because your approach to parenting is yours to mold. Are you ok with typical infant sleep patterns? Do you want to try to sleep train or schedule your infant's sleep—knowing approaches for these might be limited? And, most importantly, how will you deal with your sleep deprivation?

A Safe Space for Sleep

Nighttime is presumably when you want to sleep. Sure, you will have to get up to tend to the baby (possibly with someone's help), but you aren't going to have the same vigilance at 2:00 am that you are going to have at 9:00 am with your third cup of coffee. I used to divide the day into phases with my newborn while I was on maternity leave. Phase 1 being the morning wake-up and playtime, phase 2 being the morning nap, and phase 3 being noon. I imagine those without newborns would considering it to be the middle of their day, while I was already moving through what I considered to be deep into the afternoon. Then I would give up making up phases of the day because I could start to feel a little sad the day just kept coming. Despite the days being loooooonnnngggggg, I was better able to watch the baby during the day than in the wee hours of the morning. Because of our own circadian rhythms, when you are asleep, you want your baby's sleep area to be one in which they can't get into trouble.

What's trouble? Newborns lack head control. Many people know this, so they instinctively support the back of their infant's neck when holding them. I think the lack of head control also makes people a little reticent to hold a baby. That said, if you support the head, even if you mess up for a minute, the baby will be ok. They are not as fragile as you think. You don't want the baby's head to be in a weird position for long though. Think about what is inside your neck: your spine, your airway or trachea, and your feeding tube or esophagus. Newborns have a very tiny and more collapsible airway. So, yes, they tolerate the lack of head support for a little bit, but they need to sleep on a surface that supports their head and neck to allow them to breathe easy and keep their tiny airways open for air exchange.

Super easy, right? Well…not exactly, because infant sleep patterns are not typical and communicating with a newborn is difficult. They can't tell you when they are tired or why they woke up screaming. It's all on you to decipher the nonverbal communication they throw at you. That, and companies are not interested in helping

A Safe Sleep Space

A flat sleep surface is so important for newborns. Their head should be in line with the body without the chance of slouching over. The American Academy of Pediatrics recommends a safe sleep space. Let's discuss the 3 important tenets of safe sleep environments.

1. A flat sleep surface

2. Baby on their back

3. Nothing with them when they sleep. That means no pillows, bumpers, blankets, stuffies, lovies, or anything else.

your baby get safe sleep—they are interested in profiting off your exhaustion and anxiety. Products marketed for newborns are often not meant for sleep. Families can have a false sense of security when placing their baby for sleep in a bouncer or inclined surface that has a picture of a baby snoozing in it—and then focusing on watching TV or cooking dinner. Remember: Caring for an infant is demanding because of the high level of vigilance. To leave the baby in a space where you don't have to be watching them, you need to make sure it's a safe one for them to snooze in. Infants should always be placed on their backs to sleep. (Review the "A Safe Sleep Space" table again for the 3 tenets of safe sleep, and memorize them.) Once your baby is big enough to roll to their stomach and can also roll from their stomach to their back, and you notice they prefer to be on their belly, you don't need to constantly roll them back onto their back. Parents have told me they would run in and roll them back when they noticed the baby move on the monitor. This is not necessary; if your baby can roll both ways, they have enough body control so that being on their stomach won't block their airway. What you want to make sure is there is nothing in the crib that could block their nose or their mouth if they roll into it, and they aren't swaddled when they roll so they can be hands free.

Let's memorize the 3 important tenets of safe sleep together: on a flat surface, on their back, and alone. Why do pediatricians ask you to set up this boring sleep environment? This gets back to them and you breathing easy when you aren't watching them. Pediatricians are protective of a baby who can't control their head, and babies have those very tiny airways, or windpipes. If you investigate a baby's nose, you won't see much; their nostrils are pretty small. In addition, they like to breathe through their nose. Their tiny airway starts at their nose and goes down their neck, so you want to place them in a position to sleep that will keep their airway open for air to pass through to their lungs and eventually their bodies.

This is a good time to explain some science too. Because over many decades, excellent information has been collected showing that a safe sleep environment is protective for babies. Before the Safe to Sleep guidelines were created in the 1990s by organizations like the American Academy of Pediatrics and the National Institutes of Health, there were many more sudden unexpected infant deaths (SUIDs) or infants who died of sudden infant death syndrome (SIDS). If you are a visual person like I am, the following graph, which you can also find on the Centers for Disease Control and Prevention (CDC) website, will help illustrate this point for you:

TRENDS IN SUID RATES BY CAUSE OF DEATH, 1990–2022

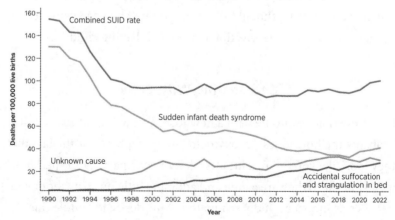

On the left-hand side of this graph you can view the number of deaths per 100,000 live births. This can be scary to think about, but death is what the CDC looks at in these cases and what prompts pediatricians to passionately educate families about when they discuss safe sleep. Within the graphic you can see the lines for SIDS and SUIDs start to fall, meaning fewer cases of SIDS and SUIDs. This happened in the mid-1990s when safe sleep guidelines came out. However, the bottommost line is slowly increasing. It refers to accidental suffocation and strangulation in bed, or ASSB. Unlike SIDS, you probably haven't heard of ASSB. While ASSB includes the words "in bed," it refers to infants dying on an unsafe sleep surface that has the potential to limit their breathing. Think couch cushions, pillows, other soft bedding, or blankets—these have been identified as the cause of suffocation for these babies. The majority of these deaths happen before 6 months of age. So, the newborn period is the time to establish safe sleep routines.

Does that mean you can never sleep with your child and should be constantly watching your infant when they sleep? No, that's not sustainable for you and won't help you build a good relationship with your baby. Your focus should be on *maintaining a safe sleep environment* and putting thought into how you will manage your sleep deprivation, as sleep deprivation comes with having children.

Bed-sharing With Baby

It is irresistible to cuddle with a newborn. You will want to do it. It's probably the hormones (ie, oxytocin—see Chapter 6) or the fact that they look like you or are a little version of your partner. Or perhaps it's just because they are a cute and adorable little human whom you perceive as innocent. It doesn't matter; your desire to cuddle this sweet baby can be strong (and if it's not—focus on the long game—

you've got a whole life to build your love). Having a newborn doing skin to skin on your chest in a frog-legged position with their little warm bodies and fast hearts—that kind of skin-to-skin contact is priceless and soothing for both of you. I'd never say "no" skin to skin with your baby.

Here's my practical advice: Don't risk bed-sharing or being in a place where when you are snuggling with a baby you might fall asleep. Being curled up on the couch with an adorable baby is asking for you both to snooze. Remember, newborns need a lot of supervision, and their parents need a lot of support. Having a family member, a friend, a hired person, or someone else there to help you doesn't mean they have to be tending to the newborn 24/7; a lot of the time they are tending to the parents, and you deserve that. Some people might be happy doing laundry or helping with meal prep or dishes, but even just watching you while you cuddle your baby on the couch is a true gift. That way, if you do fall asleep, someone is there to make sure you and your baby stay safe. Help comes in many forms; *just being there is one of them.*

In my bed I sleep with 2 pillows, a regular sheet that I turn into a twisty sheet when tossing and turning, and a fun patterned comforter. None of these items are safe for a baby. You should not bed-share with your baby. You might be thinking this is hard, and you are correct—but it is something you can control to make a safer sleep environment for your baby. The American Academy of Pediatrics recommends that parents and babies sleep in the same room but on separate sleep surfaces, ideally for the first 6 months. Other things you can control are not smoking or drinking excessively before you care for your infant. (A sober parent is much less likely to fall asleep and roll onto their baby.) If you are taking any medications that might make you sleepy, being the only person available to care for your baby at nighttime or when you take them might not be the best decision. Pediatricians will tell you not to have your baby in the bed with you. That said, talk openly and honestly with your pediatrician about the reality of what you're doing. Your pediatrician should be someone who is going to answer your questions honestly. Your story will also be impactful by educating them on how to respond to other parents who might be having similar sleep struggles. I am always learning from families and find their experiences enlightening. Sharing stories is such an important way for everyone to learn and grow together.

When I have parents who bed-share I counsel them to strip the bed down to just the mattress and a fitted sheet that fits directly over the mattress. That way the bed is way less comfortable so the chances of you snoozing soundly go down. This does not mean I say sleep with your baby—because bed-sharing again is not something I recommend. If you want to be close to your baby while you sleep, place them in a separate safe sleep environment (on their back, flat surface, nothing else with them) that is close to you. That way you can comfort them at arm's length in the middle of the night and have their physical presence next to you. The most cost-effective option might be a play yard set up next to your bed. For my babies we used a play crib that was easy to move and set up in the space next to my bed and the wall. There are also small bassinets that you can buy to insert next to you—though I found they were expensive and fleeting as you couldn't use them when baby started to grow bigger. Another more pricey option is a co-sleeper that attaches to your bed; you can't fit in it, but the baby does. In addition it can be more expensive and difficult to attach—so ensure the co-sleeper is placed properly before using it. You don't need anything fancy, just a flat surface baby can lie in on their back with nothing else around them except you at arm's-length away.

Your infant will appreciate that closeness for many months, but if it's too much for you after a while, move them to a place where you can address their needs easily—but keep it in the same room. Recommendations on safe sleep and general infant care advise you to have the baby in the room with you for at least the first 6 months after birth, so you are readily available to address any concerns they might have. Interestingly, some parents balk at not being able to bedshare, but then also balk at needing to have their baby in the room with them for several months. Listen, we aren't going to perform every recommendation perfectly. It's protection over perfection we try to emphasize. Around 90% of sudden infant deaths occur within the first 6 months. So for all 3 of my babies I dedicated those 6 months to room sharing. With my first baby she was out of the room right when that SIDS risk dropped; for my other 2 they lasted 10 and 9 months, respectively, in a room next to me. It's important to be near your newborn and young baby when they sleep—so make this proximity a goal.

If you are really hoping a great night's sleep is in your future with your baby and you envision bed-sharing as the best way for them to sleep...there are actually studies showing bed-sharing decreases the length and quality of sleep for everyone involved. It might seem easier, but it's not giving either of you the space to rest. I am going to offer you a snapshot of how I slept last night with my oldest 2 children. I never allowed my kids to sleep with me as newborns and for the first year of their lives. But my strict control over that led to a lax response to them entering my bed as they grew older. Doing so in the newborn period is not safe and you don't want to jeopardize those *years* of sleeping together if it's something you have dreamt about. Honestly, though, sleeping with a young kid is not all it's cracked up to be. Here is a timeline of the incredible sleep I got while pregnant with my third child.

8:00 pm: I put them to bed in their own rooms.

8:45 pm: Both my son and daughter left their rooms in an attempt to escape sleep.

8:47 pm: I walked them back to their beds. Tucked them in, explained in my serious tone that it was time to go to bed. Mommy is not herself without good sleep and we sleep better in our own spaces.

10:30 pm: Feeling like I'd done a great job of keeping them in their beds and after some mommy "me time" I fell asleep.

3:00 am: I was woken up by my son sitting on my face and then snuggling in bed on top of me. He whispered something about chocolate milk, or maybe that was just in a dream. Distressed at the early wake-up time, I tried to move over to make space for him to sleep next to me and not on top, only to find my daughter had snuck into the bed (hour unknown) and was on the other side of me. My kids are quite wiggly. I am now trapped between the wiggles.

3:20 am: I found myself walking down the hallway and decided to sleep in my daughter's room. It was the first room I came to. I climbed into her bed.

3:40 am: My son didn't find this acceptable, followed me, and climbed in the twin bed with me. I decided to go back to my bed, but my son wasn't asleep yet and screamed for me. Deliriously tired and body aching, I now engaged my husband to deal with my son (in my daughter's room) and fell back asleep with my daughter in my own bed.

5:00 am: My daughter woke up ready to start her day. In frustration, I sternly encouraged (read whisper yelled) her to lie down.

6:00 am: My son returns, again on my face.

6:30 am: I am now awake, so we all got up despite my alarm being set for 7:00 am.

Suffice to say, glorious nights of sleep with your children await you after the newborn period. I would argue my situation is slightly worse than dealing with a newborn who has a set list of wants, as opposed to a strong and illogical desire to drink chocolate milk at 3:00 am. But it's not just about placing a baby for sleep in a safe space, it's also about making sure you can maintain that space throughout the night. To be the parent you want to be involves some degree of feeling rested so you have the bandwidth to actually parent. There is so much focus on infant sleep because, while we have some descriptions of how newborns sleep, each baby is an individual and their sleep is going to change based on so many factors. But it will change. Your needs aren't going to change that much; you'll want those 6 to 8 hours of sleep, but your newborn, infant, toddler, and even preschooler won't have the same notions of how to rest and relax. So, you are going to have to adapt, be creative, and have a plan in place to tolerate sleep deprivation. Here is a graph of typical sleep hours as kids grow:

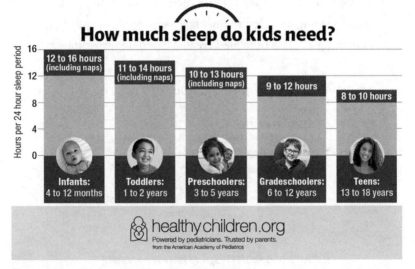

The American Academy of Pediatrics (AAP) has issued a statement of endorsement supporting these guidelines from the American Academy of Sleep Medicine (AASM).

Source: American Academy of Pediatrics. Healthy sleep habits: how many hours does your child need? HealthyChildren.org. Accessed June 14, 2024. https://www.healthychildren.org/English/healthy-living/sleep/Pages/healthy-sleep-habits-how-many-hours-does-your-child-need.aspx and *J Clin Sleep Med.* 2016;12(6):785–786.

Sleep Train, or Refrain?

Newborns don't sleep through the night. Sleep changes during infancy and even into the early years of children's lives. You aren't going to know exactly when it is going to change. Parents love to guess at exactly what their baby will do, instead of listening to their baby, gauging their temperament, and being content to allow the baby to take the lead on their needs. Sleep may be a time for active observation (akin to active listening) instead of trying to predict what kind of sleeper your kid might be. For those into prediction, I've heard families attempt to estimate periods of time when their infant's sleep might change and refer to these changes as growth spurts, frequency days, or wonder weeks. These are times when a baby seems fussier and more animated and might need more attention from their parents. In truth, though, babies always need a lot of attention. If you read about all these catchy phrases and create a timeline for when your infant might experience a growth spurt, a period of intensive feeding, or a developmental kaleidoscope of emotion, it will look something like this timeline I created based on my readings:

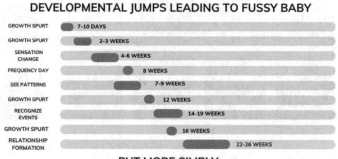

DEVELOPMENTAL JUMPS LEADING TO FUSSY BABY

GROWTH SPURT	7-10 DAYS
GROWTH SPURT	2-3 WEEKS
SENSATION CHANGE	4-6 WEEKS
FREQUENCY DAY	8 WEEKS
SEE PATTERNS	7-9 WEEKS
GROWTH SPURT	12 WEEKS
RECOGNIZE EVENTS	14-19 WEEKS
GROWTH SPURT	16 WEEKS
RELATIONSHIP FORMATION	22-26 WEEKS

PUT MORE SIMPLY:
BABY (< 6 MONTHS) + FUSSY = ANYTIME.

Data were derived from Australian Breastfeeding Association. Fussy periods. Updated April 2022. Accessed November 7, 2024. https://www.breastfeeding.asn.au/resources/fussy-periods; KellyMom. Growth spurts. Updated August 16, 2023. Accessed November 7, 2024. https://kellymom.com/hot-topics/growth-spurts; The Wonder Weeks. *The Wonder Weeks book*. Accessed November 7, 2024. https://thewonderweeks.com/the-wonder-weeks-book.

It's any time during the first 6 months after birth. Is this surprising? No, because only 40% of infants (fewer than half) are actually "sleeping through the night" at 6 months old. Your baby could be fussy for so many reasons—growth, development, hunger, a dirty diaper, a cold hand, being aggravated by a button on their onesie, a bad smell—you get my point. They are constantly developing and adapting to their environment, and the only thing certain about an infant is they *will* change. Many parents feel exhausted keeping up with the change in development that is a hallmark of infancy. It leads some to feel frustrated that they can't get a grasp on who their baby is—and how to make them sleep. That said, you will likely get a sense of their personality in the newborn period. It's just that their brains are growing so fast that they can barely keep up with themselves. If you are looking to find a book or an app that will tell you with certainty what your baby is going to be doing in 6 weeks, you won't find it. But as a parent, I get the desperate need to feel like you have some control and some understanding of your infant. It's incredibly hard to take a step back and just learn from them.

That's where sleep training comes in. The name implies you can teach them a thing or two about nodding off, which sounds excellent, and more and more people are doing it. This is especially true in the United States where our work schedules do not align with our needs or our child's needs.

So, should you, like many other parents, sleep train your baby? Let's take a look at sleep training to decide. All types of sleep training require some sort of behavioral modification—or trying to control and change your behaviors to influence how the baby sleeps or otherwise behaves. Remember, infant sleep looks different depending on the baby, and there is a large variation in what typical sleep for a newborn is. So, already, sleep training can't be the same for every infant. That said, the most common way we try to modulate infant behavior is by extinction interventions—things like crying it out. Crying it out consists of telling your baby they are going to bed, putting them in a crib, and letting them cry until they fall asleep. With these methods, the belief is that the parent's attention reinforces a bad behavior—like crying. So, remove the parent's attention, and the baby can figure it out and learn how to self-soothe. This method might just leave a baby wailing in a closed-off room with a parent wondering if that is ok.

Some people worry the baby will be scarred by the sleep training, that it is a trauma for them. I'm less worried about that and more focused on the fact that your baby needs you. Crying is a baby's way of telling you that and communicating their needs (see Chapter 8). And sure, it's ok to not meet your baby's needs every second of every day, but if you are letting them cry it out for long periods of time, what lesson are you teaching them? That their main form of communication is a failure? How is it shaping their brain? These questions are unanswerable but ones I think about as a pediatrician.

It's these kinds of questions that ultimately have led to other methods of crying it out; they include checking in on the baby after a short period of time, then slowly stretching that time interval until they stop crying and fall asleep. Some recommend a method in which you stay in the room until the baby falls asleep, not touching or holding them, just being there for them. I think these methods are kinder and allow for more 2-way communication. If you want to raise an empathetic child who responds to the emotions of others, you have to find ways to be responsive to the baby when they need you. Not when a book tells you they might need you because of some developmental spurt, but when the baby actually tells you they do. It's good not to ignore them or struggle with not responding to them when it's what you both want. Be true to the qualities you want to have as a parent and those you want your baby to have. I've often caught myself saying "little kid, little problems," but for the baby being left alone in a room to figure it out by themselves, it is a big deal. Especially if they don't have the temperament of a "figure-it-out" type of kid.

Does that mean I am against sleep training? No. I can take it or leave it. I think of crying as communication and not a form of trauma. Besides, sleep training a newborn is not truly possible.

Newborns change week to week as their brains expand and their bodies grow. They also need to eat every 2 to 4 hours, as they don't have the fat and glucose or sugar stores to maintain their metabolism. Some proponents of sleep training recommend starting as early as 6 weeks. That sounds almost impossible to me—actually training a baby who doesn't even have a grasp on sleep and wake cycles. I'd say wait until age 6 months if you really want a baby to learn. Consistency with any training is key. So that means you must be committed to your choice. What I've decided to be committed to is my relationship with the child. Recognizing they are individuals and training myself to engage with and listen to them. You don't get to choose the person they will be; parenting is the chaotic pleasure of loving the person you've got.

To formally sleep train an infant who isn't fully cognizant of their surroundings and your teachings is a challenge. They aren't going to sleep on the schedule you want them to, and they don't understand that they are supposed to do what you ask of them. Infants read our body language and adapt their responses to the environment we create. If sleep training makes you upset and frustrated, that might derail your attempts to get the baby to relax and snooze. Because a baby who sees or feels their caregiver being riled up is not going to settle down; they are going to feel distressed alongside you.

If sleep training is going to make you happy and you are going to be calm and collected every time you address your crying baby, maybe sleep training is for you. If you can't model your best self in a practice that will take nights of dedication and intervention, you need a new plan. Consider this: You are asking your baby to find a way to self-soothe and not rely on your always being around. This is a noble goal because you are *everything* to your newborn and to your growing baby. The sun, moon, stars, planets, and far-reaching galaxies. Asking them not to rely on you is against their very nature. They *need* you. Some babies might be ready for the challenge, but many aren't going to be soothed except by the people they love and trust in a dark nighttime world. What I do worry about is this: As the electricity flows through their exponentially growing brains, they are building circuitry, and how you react to them will ultimately influence their response to the world. Sure, it might teach them independence, and this might be an important value to you. But just know that that's the lesson you are teaching. If empathy is also important to you, then intervening in some way as you train might be beneficial to the person you are raising. You need to begin to understand the qualities you think are important to impart to your child from a very young age. At the end of a long day, give yourself and the baby some grace; there are other ways to deal with sleep deprivation than sleep training.

TOOLS TO SELF-SOOTHE

There are ways to deal with infant sleep issues that don't involve trying to train them.

1. **Create a nighttime ritual.** Don't feed the baby right before bed. Feed them, then change their diaper, and start reading a book. Consider an activity like massage or a soothing song before putting them down. We used to use an unscented, uncolored lotion on my first daughter and massage her arms and legs right after her bath and before sliding her into her footie PJs. I was always jealous of her nighttime massages. I rewrote the lyrics to Juvenile's song *Slow Motion* and would sing "rub lotion on me" as we went through our routine.

2. **Consider a pacifier.** If you are breastfeeding—establish a good latch and make sure baby is starting to gain weight and then introduce a pacifier. If you are not directly feeding at the breast—introduce that pacifier whenever you like. I've had friends who are vehemently against pacifier use because of concerns for pacifier addiction later. I am pro-pacifier and am not sure you can label an infant an addict if they like one. Some babies just really love to suck; it soothes them. Also, there are good data to suggest pacifier use can help prevent sudden

---

infant death syndrome (SIDS). Yes, you might need to wean your toddler off one in the future, but a happy sleepy baby who can use a pacifier to self-soothe is, in my opinion, worth it.

3. **Try swaddles**. Babies don't have well-developed nervous systems and will kick their arms and legs at random, punching themselves in the face or startling themselves awake. My last baby had really long hair that she loved to pull and then became so confused when it hurt her. A swaddle keeps them contained, like they were in the womb. Swaddles should never be weighted, so that infants can move and breath comfortably and not overheat. They also shouldn't be used in older babies who can move around more and roll, so most swaddling must be discontinued when baby begins to roll, which is generally around 4 months old. But for a newborn they might provide a relaxing squeeze. I remember once putting my baby girl in a swaddle, placing her in my bed as I put on a shirt, and watching as she gently faceplanted into the lumpy sheets strewn on my mattress. It was just for a second, but it was enough to scare me for half a day. I saw how a little baby could get into trouble by being unable to move on an unsafe sleep surface. So, make sure to swaddle in your boring, box-like bassinet without anything that could tip the baby over. Worried about hips in a swaddle? Your concern is not unfounded, and tightly wrapping the hips could affect their development. There are swaddles that allow the hips to move more freely and just provide a snug fit over the shoulders and chest. I prefer those swaddles. And don't stress if you can't swaddle a baby like the postpartum nurse. Any good postpartum nurse can swaddle a baby in a napkin and make it look easy. It is not easy. As a fumbling doctor, I have swaddled hundreds of babies in hospital blankets. About 70% of the time, I can get something that looks nice and snug, but about 30% of the time the baby escapes my swaddle. That's why I recommend hook-and-loop fasteners, Velcro, or button swaddles to all new families. Fewer user errors!

4. **Embrace daytime naps.** Often for infants, sleep begets more sleep. If they spend the day snoozing and don't get overtired, they are less likely to be tired and strung out at bedtime. And never feel guilty about holding them all day. This is how you

learn what a tired baby looks like, the cues that means they need a nap. Yawning, eye rubbing, droopy eyelids—time to start that sleep routine!

5. **Look for signs of drowsiness.** Holding, feeding and snuggling your baby are wonderful and help them feel drowsy. When you start to recognize your baby is going to fall asleep—try placing them on a safe sleep surface while still a little bit awake. This will allow them time to get used to falling asleep alone in a safe sleep space after getting the incredible feeling of your attention and focus.

I wish I had a magical sleep solution for you. Something that always works for every baby. What I want you to take away from this chapter is that babies aren't programmed to sleep through the night. Forcing them to do so doesn't mean they won't wake up and have periods of poor sleep. What's important is making going to sleep a calm and relaxing experience for your baby as opposed to stressful. Come up with a nighttime routine that is enjoyable and stick to it, one that makes everyone feel happy. Sleep helps with bonding because getting sleep makes you feel more in control and in touch with your emotions.

Your Sleep(less) Survival Guide

With a baby, you are not afforded a day off. The sleep deprivation didn't catch me in the first week after having a newborn, but by the second week I was dragging. And I felt horrible because, what was I doing? I wasn't helping to save lives like I usually did at my job as a baby doctor. I was just keeping a healthy one going. But this is such an important job; so for everyone keeping a baby happy and healthy, celebrate the hard work you are doing. For me, anxiety and borderline depression crept in as the stretches of sleep I used to enjoy thinned out. My sleep became an abstract stringing together of an hour or 2 of sleep interrupted by the sheep-like bleating of a newborn's cry. Despite my adrenaline filled night spent working in the hospital, I had never been so sleepy.

This exhaustion is what drives parents to want to sleep train or spend hundreds of dollars on an unproven sleep gadget for their infant. Desperately trying to ignore typical infant physiology to find a chunk of time to slumber. But I advise you not to do that. So how do you sleep better with a baby?

Dealing With the Deprivation

Realize that just because you need uninterrupted stretches of sleep, your infant doesn't. How can you get to sleep?

Work on your sleep hygiene. That phone you love to scroll while feeding the baby or lying in bed? Put it outside the room. I took to charging my phone at night on a different floor of the house. Switch to a traditional alarm clock if you are using your phone as one, and turn off the electronics a half hour or so before going to bed. That includes the television. If you have a TV in your bedroom, take it out now. Banish any screens from your bedroom. Beds are for sleep and baby making, not for channel surfing or streaming app hopping. Plus, television keeps you awake. You might think watching your favorite episode of *RuPaul's Drag Race* is just the kind of entertainment that will help clear your brain. But the blue light from screens tells your brain not to produce melatonin, so you are less likely to fall asleep if you are watching TV in bed. When using an alarm clock, make sure you can't easily see the numbers on it. I dim my electronic alarm clock to an almost invisible state. I hide the time because when I see that I've woken up at 4:00 am and only have 2 more hours to sleep before my kid wakes up and finds me, I'm much less likely to sleep those 2 hours. I'm likely to fret about how I won't sleep, or the things I must do, or how overwhelmed I am. Life with a newborn is timeless, so embrace the lack of a structured day.

If you need some technology surrounding you, consider a fan or a white noise machine. Some sound device that lulls you into an unconscious state and cuts the edge of other noises in the room like the baby shuffling or heavy breathing. I'm not saying to make it so loud you don't hear the baby; I'm just saying that if your baby is in a safe sleep space next to you and you've made sure to put them in a worry-free position you can slightly muffle the sounds they emit because babies are fitful sleepers. White noise is good to lull you to sleep. You will have nighttime awakenings, and you can shut off the white noise in the wee hours of the morning if you don't want it going all night.

This is also the time for you to do some rituals. Take time to really create your bedtime routine. I like to shower at night; the sound of the water and feeling clean help me cuddle up in the sheets. Then I brush my teeth, futz with my hair, and read a book. Right before I go to sleep—because I can't jettison my devices so easily—I cue up a 10-minute meditation and lie on the bed just breathing in and out, trying to follow my breath. Full disclosure: Quieting my mind doesn't seem to ever happen. But it puts my body in a restful state. I dim my bedside alarm clock and try to clock out. This might not be your routine, but here's a summary of things that might help soothe you.

- Set a bedtime that is the same every night; routine will soothe you in the out-of-control newborn period.
- Shut off your devices, get your TV out of the room. I said to do it a half hour or so before bed, but some people need a few hours to wind down.

- Think about a light snack or a bedtime tea. I've just about become addicted to rooibos tea before bed. It's a South African bush tea you can let steep forever and has a sweet and caramelly finish.
- Take a shower or a warm bath.
- Consider mindful meditation to at least try to calm your brain.
- Read a book, preferably a boring one. Try rereading one of the classics like *Moby Dick*; a discussion of what type of whale harpoon you might have used in the 1800s is one of the reasons I have never finished the book. It finishes me and I have fallen asleep reading it.
- Listen to something calming like white noise or a nice slow song.

Your bedtime routine doesn't have to exclude your baby. It can incorporate them. Newborns will probably go to bed when you do, and if it's an older baby or a toddler, start earlier and slip into your own routine when they go down. They can take a shower with you if there is room, practice meditation with you, read with you; my newborns were well versed in literature that put us both to sleep in the postpartum period. And what baby doesn't love a good calming melody? Make bedtime a routine for everyone. Remember, your children will emulate you, so if you show them the importance of sleep habits early on, at some point they will rub off (here's looking at your teenage years).

Chapter 8

I'm Not Crying, You're Crying…But Why?

t started around 6 o'clock each night. She would begin to stir, kicking her arms and legs and getting fussy and unsettled. Next came the crying. Every evening, we knew this would happen, and my husband and I would brace ourselves. Even though we anticipated it, there was no preventing it. Whatever developmental leap or bound she was taking at 6 weeks was not to be trifled with. Despite the knowledge she was about to lose it and whatever we did seemed not to matter, we still had to do something. We couldn't just let her cry. So, we went through our crying checklist. Was she fed? Burped? Changed? Check, check, check. Time to get more nuanced. I would get driven so far down my cry checklist I'd be searching for elusive hair tourniquets on her fingers and toes. I've always had long hair and a hair tourniquet is when your hair gets wrapped around a digit and cuts off blood flow to it. Maybe that was causing her pain? I never found one. Her basic needs seemed to have been met but she still wailed. And that's when, as a parent, I had a choice. I could succumb to my parental anxiety and cry too, because I couldn't help her, and my hormones wanted me to let loose. I went with this option a few times, using my baby as a teacher and finding that a good cry can be a great release. Often though I would buckle down, determined to ride out the waves of tears, letting her calm down before my breakdown began.

One song helped me through it. The Phantom of the Opera *debuted on Broadway in 1988. This '80s smash hit was one of the first Broadway shows I'd ever seen growing up in the Long Island suburbs outside New York City. I returned to it many times in my life, the songs continuing to inspire me. The meaning of those songs changes over time. For me, in my daughter's infancy, "The Point of No Return" would usher me in shuffled steps around our Philadelphia city row-home. At this point in the play, the Phantom has locked his crush (read: obsession) in the basement with him; it's one of the final acts in the play. There is no coming back from his expression of love. Swaying around the room with my inconsolable baby was for me a heightened expression of my love for her in those moments. Having children has altered every love song for me.*

Sting's "Every Breath You Take" comes to mind as another song I listened to and now makes me think about my kids growing up. Tell me you can watch your kid learning how to walk and not let those lyrics wash over your consciousness. It is a song about a creeper, but as a parent that's kind of what you are. A stalwart observer of the beginning of a life. I really needed songs to connect with when my children were newborns. Because I could never avoid getting emotional when my infant was crying; the sobs cut me to the core. So, letting my babies sit and cry on their own wasn't going to work for me. Dancing around the room to Andrew Lloyd Webber or rock superstar Sting, that's what got me through the lows.

When your baby's crying reaches the point of no return, you will work to comfort them and yourself in whatever way is needed.

Baby's First Bawl

When I am in the delivery room awaiting the appearance of my patient, their cry is the sweetest. Piercing the frenetic energy of the delivery room with an ear-splitting sound that maybe only a neo-natologist really appreciates. It is the way the baby announces their entrance to the world. Filling their lungs with air for the first time and bursting onto the scene. A quiet baby without the appropriate zeal to puff up their chest and start providing oxygen to their body worries me. That's a baby I will coax into gulping cries on the warmer. Typical techniques that make a baby squeal—and not in a cute way—are flicking their feet or running your fingers down their spine. That first cry is so important for them to transition from a life in amniotic fluid to one on dry land.

Crying Babies and Birth Parent Bodies

Crying is distressing for parents. Adults do not cry as much as babies because they have different ways of expressing themselves. Their body language and words can express sadness sometimes more than tears can. For a baby, crying is the way. This is how they signal distress. The distress could be minor: I don't like being held in this position, or the wet pee makes me feel yucky. Or it could be that they are hungry, cold, or tired.

A baby's cry is meant to elicit a response from the parent, as it is related to milk letdown. Hormonal cues flood the brain with one hormone: oxytocin. Oxytocin is the cuddliest of hormones because it helps with milk letdown and with bonding. Oxytocin makes you want to respond to your baby's cry.

I've heard parents talk about not wanting to spoil their infants and wanting them to get used to crying. The term *greedy* gets used in reference to infants a lot in the hospitals I work in. I can imagine how hard it must be for parents to feel societal pressure not to hold while the biological pull is coaxing them to pick up the baby and soothe them. But there is no way to overindulge a baby. A baby does not know they are asking to be picked up; they are signaling their needs and asking for attention and closeness. Remember, they are not trying to monopolize your time to annoy you. They are doing it because they must; their brain development depends on you.

To grow into an emotionally mature, stable, and independent adult, a baby needs one loving caregiver who addresses their needs. Someone who is attentive and responds to them. It's true that if you don't respond to a crying baby, they will eventually tire out, and if you don't respond every single time, that's ok. But if you do respond, it is not teaching your baby to be soft and needy. It is showing your infant they can depend on someone, that someone has their back. Their relationship with a loving caregiver shapes the hormones and neuronal connections of their brains. It is their everything.

Do not feel like you are spoiling your baby when you respond to their cries. As they get older, they can begin to learn to self-soothe and regulate, but when they are newborns, they need you. Their brain needs you. And you can never hold them enough.

Kinds of Cries

If you spend time listening to your baby cry, you will realize that not all cries are the same. While they can't tell you how they are feeling, the pitch and frequency of their cry may be an indication of their needs. According to research from the University of California, Los Angeles, there are 3 main types of cries: fussiness, anger, or pain. Of course, the spectrum of crying is more varied than this. Fussiness could mean that the baby needs a diaper change or is hungry, but this cry is going to sound different from that of a baby who is overly emotional and now angry about their situation. You can download the researchers' app to help you interpret cries.

However, I don't think you need an app. I think you just need to know that it is possible to interpret and understand your infant's cries. If you start to systematically work through the possible reasons for their crying, you might be able to determine what the cry is about over time. You are training the baby to be in the world, and they are training you to understand their world. That's relationship building at its finest.

When the crying happens, reflect on your day. Does the crying usually happen in the evening? (Most parents report the hours of 6:00 pm to 12:00 am can be a real tearjerker.) Is there something that sparks it or is it fun and spontaneous like the date nights you used to have? (Of note, I knew a couple who once got completely ready to go to the movies, then realized they had a baby and someone needed to be home for that baby. In that moment they realized going to the movies was no longer something they could do without child care). You are looking for patterns, not to diagnose your baby with anything.

Babies cry. Often, a baby's stomach gets blamed for the crying; they are gassy or they spit up a lot. Pay attention to that, but also look to see if your baby cries after seeming to have periods of happiness or peace. They probably do. You are a baby watcher now, so take notes if you need to, but chances are your baby isn't plagued by something you need to fix. Because, well, babies cry. This is how they communicate with you.

Find out what works for your baby. What worked for your neighbor's baby might work for yours. What worked for the Instagram celebrity's baby almost certainly will not work for yours. This is your baby. Only you and baby are working hard on the relationship you are building. Anyone outside of your relationship isn't really going to know what works for you. I don't get it, they don't get it, you truly get it. But here are some things that might help.

THE CRY BABY CHECKLIST

What can you do if your baby is crying? Checklist time! You need a crying toolkit to address their unspoken needs before you reach the point of no return and succumb to swaying, mumbling, and some form of prayer to wait for the baby to relax. If you do these things, you can be confident you have covered most of the baby's basic needs.

Feed the baby. Has it been over 2 hours since the baby's last bottle of milk or moment on the breast? If it hasn't been quite that amount of time, I'd say try some of the suggestions below, but babies like a full belly and need to feed around 8 to 12 times in a 24-hour period. So think about feeding the baby.

Pacify your love. If you've read any other part of this book, you know I am generally pro-pacifier. If you've fed the baby, and your baby is a sucker, try a pacifier.

Check the diaper. No one, including your baby, likes to sit in their own pee or poop. Ok, my toddler seemed totally content to run around in their own poop for hours instead of learning how to use the potty—but toddlers are a different beast. This is your newborn; they don't want to feel dirty. Change them.

My gosh, put on some clothes! Sometimes just being too warm or too cold can set a baby off. Again, I don't live in your house. If I did, the house would be at 68 °F on the dot, and the moment it got to 70 °F, there would be sweating and cursing. This is my rule of thumb for temperatures for babies: however you feel in what you are wearing, the baby probably needs one more layer than you. If you are totally comfortable in a T-shirt and shorts, the baby probably just needs a cotton long-sleeve onesie. If you are super cold and bundled up in a sweater with some teeth chatter, consider a short-sleeved onesie underneath a fleece long-sleeve onesie for your baby. And as you can tell, I adore a good onesie. Preferably one with zippers because the snaps are a cry catalyst for all parents that have to fasten them.

Stimulation. For periods of the day your baby will want to be awake with you. Looking at you with their intense baby stare and as you dangle toys in their face. A typical day might be spent in the house, but on some days you might be out and about with loud noises, lots of people, and lots to put a baby's developing nervous system into high gear. If you feel stressed after a long and busy day, the baby might too. Time for a dark room or a walk in the woods with the stroller.

This is boring. Maybe you have been in a dark room or the quiet woods all day. Your baby might be saying it's time for some fun. Consider some play with toys or a walk outside in the daylight.

Swaddling. Probably everyone's greatest trauma they don't remember is having to leave the womb. Babies really enjoy being swaddled. You heard me talk about how this isn't a forever thing; around age 4 months they could start to roll and then swaddles are a no-go. But sometimes tucking them into a nice swaddle is what they really need to calm down. No more flailing arms and legs, they surrender to the sweet womb-like wonder of a nice tight squeeze.

White noise toys. Speaking of the womb, it's not this quiet place where the baby lies in a dark, soundless void. When you are pregnant, you are carrying that baby through your life. Cars on the street, chatting with your loved ones, listening to music at an overpriced concert. Likely, your abdominal muscles and skin muffle the sounds a bit, but they reach your growing baby. Not to mention there is a lot of blood flowing around the baby. The placenta is probably pretty quiet (love you placenta), but there are major arteries feeding your uterus that hum around the baby night and day. So, it's no wonder that white noise—the drumming of a heartbeat or the drone of a fan—can really help soothe your baby. After all, this isn't a quiet world we live in. Remember to try to keep the noise low, and shut it off when the baby is calm. Loud noises can affect hearing, and you want to use soft soothing noises to calm; then once you've achieved your goal, silence might be more soothing.

Take a walk. Sometimes babies just want to be with you. Consider carrying the baby around the block or around the house as you do chores. Or put them in a stroller and literally stroll. You don't need a destination when you have a crying baby; plus it's a little exercise for you. When caring for a newborn, every little bit counts! And remember, strolling can also be a womb-like activity because the baby literally walked around with their birth parent for nearly 10 months. So sashay your way into having a happy baby.

Docking station. Sometimes holding onto a crying baby can be too much. That is why the baby industrial complex has created swings, walking mimickers, and vibrating mats to help you soothe your baby. Remember, any angled device is not for sleeping, but I swore by a nonmechanical baby hammock I could rock with my foot to soothe my baby in times of fussiness. Having a safe place to put down the baby that will rock, sway, or jiggle them gently into calmness is often a needed respite for a parent.

None of this is working. Your advice is awful. I'm burning this book.

You've done it all. Every single trick in this book. You are frustrated, tired, and upset, so how are you going to take care of this crying baby?

Before you burn this book, which honestly could be cathartic, remember that babies will cry. If the typical soothing strategies don't work, talk to your pediatrician. Bring your log or observations of the baby crying and explore if the baby really isn't feeling well or if the milk you are giving them isn't sitting right. Crying counseling is in the wheelhouse of every pediatrician, because excessive infant crying sucks.

You've probably noticed that not once in this cry chapter has the word colic been mentioned. I don't think colic is a helpful diagnosis because it lends itself to pathologizing what might be normal baby activity. Because, again, babies do cry to communicate. The technical definition of colic is when an infant cries excessively. This crying takes place in the first 3 months, occurs more than 3 days a week, and lasts for more than 3 hours. There are also claims the colic cry is different, that it sounds like a pain cry, and the infant genuinely looks uncomfortable. Maybe they are grimacing, pale in color, or stiffening and arching while they wail. Crying, though, is always kind of ugly. I'm not sure even the most adorable infant could make crying seem attractive.

The other thing is when babies cry a lot, and we put the name colic to it, there is no treatment or remedy for colic. Thus, we might be missing a bigger issue. With colic, parents will ask about medications like simethicone or things like gripe water to soothe the baby's belly. I caution against overmedicating a baby (simethicone in my experience acts like a placebo) or giving them anything but a type of milk. This diagnosis also makes families feel they must take a hard look at their feeding of the baby—an already emotionally charged area. Are they doing it too much and overfeeding? Does the breastfeeding parent need to eliminate foods from their diet (eg, eggs, wheat, nuts [emphasis on the nuts, as it can be difficult to do elimination diets]) to make sure some food sensitivity isn't the cause? These are things you might try, but again the first thing to do is talk to your pediatrician. Because we just don't know what causes colic. We don't know if it's just overstimulation from being in a new world, or having too much gas because the baby's young intestines are still trying to figure out their coordinated movements, or if the baby is just one who swallowed a ton of air because they are a baby, a baby who loves to cry.

For a baby who cries excessively, pediatricians will want to see them in the office. That starts with your pediatrician listening to you, actively listening. The stories a parent tells about their children are usually the first step in diagnosis. Your pediatrician should be someone with whom you can be open and honest about your baby's habits and what you have been trying to do to soothe them. Then there is the physical exam, which usually starts with taking the baby's vital signs. Do they have a high heart rate for some reason? Is there a fever? Infection may be an emergency to be dealt with in the moment. The full physical exam might turn up some source of discomfort, like a hernia or a protrusion of the bowel into the labia majora or into the scrotum. It might uncover a cut on the anus (called a fissure) or maybe (a fear of mine) a hair tourniquet. Examining babies from head to toe is essential, so any physical issue can be ruled out. However, in cases of colic, only around 5% of babies will be given a diagnosis to explain the constant crying. That means for 95% of crying babies there will not be a known cause.

It comes down to finding reassurance that your baby is doing something a lot of babies do. Crying is their "jam" even though the sound and force of it can feel like a wham.

If you haven't already torched this book, there are 2 important things you need to know.

1. You are a good parent; having a crying baby doesn't make you a bad one.
2. This is not *who* your baby is, but for a newborn this is *what* a baby does.

Of course, you feel insecure when your baby cries nonstop at night and you can't comfort them. This is a reasonable feeling. Sure, you are living with the sensation that you've lost control and generally are bad at parenting. Feelings of inadequacy make you human. They will push you to discover new things about your baby, but they shouldn't cripple you into thinking you cannot parent. Your relationship with this little human is just beginning and babies change every week. You will see nuggets of the human you are going to raise, love, and bond with—a baby is not the sum of their cries.

Which gets to the *who* of your baby. When the baby is wailing and you are struggling, the love you want to feel for this person will be challenged. You'll wonder if you just got the bad baby, the fussy baby, and this is now your lot in life. Do not judge a baby by their crying in the first few weeks after birth. Their behavior while they are trying to figure out the world is not who they are. The fun and cool reality about parenting is, in a world where we have little control, you get to influence who this baby will become. In many ways, how you plan your responses to and respite from the baby's crying says more about you than the baby. Try to channel some of that worry into your hopes and dreams about how you want to parent. Being introspective can be difficult when someone is flipping out next to you, but those moments can be a time for reflection. A time to go back to the vision board you made and dance around it (hey, you've reached the point of no return anyway) to realize this is a long game and you are just at the starting line. So if you expend all your energy running circles at the starting line, you aren't putting time into training for the marathon. Building a loving relationship with an infant takes time, focus, and listening in ways you might not have before. With your ears, sure, but also with your other senses so you get to know the little human in front of you.

Chapter 9

Eat, Sleep, Poop, Build Exponential Neuronal Networks, Repeat

orking in the neonatal intensive care unit (NICU) of a large children's hospital can be described in one word: intense. The infants there are ill, having traveled from across the country for specialized care or for the hope of an experimental treatment. Many have chronic diagnoses that will follow them throughout their lives and require the support of many different types of pediatricians.

On this particular morning, we were doing walking rounds and at the bedside of a baby who had suffered severe brain damage at birth. Their brain development overall was in question. The medical team feared the baby might not be able to do the things we take for granted, like eating on their own. Then there are questions about the baby's future. Will they be able to go to school? Participate in sports? Build meaningful relationships? A baby's brain has the capacity to heal more than an adult's after an injury, but by how much? There were a lot of unknowns.

On this day we were focused on the baby's nutrition. The baby had a tube going from their nose to stomach to provide the milk they needed to grow. We call this a naso (nose) gastric (stomach) tube, or an NG tube for short. Sucking is a reflex newborns have, but this baby had not yet exhibited it. There was still hope the baby could practice feeding and gain the skills needed to go home without any type of tube. We were also worried the baby might need something called a gastrostomy tube, or G-tube, which is placed into the stomach and sticks out of the belly to supply milk directly into the gut.

*The baby's mother was cradling her baby while deftly propping
a cell phone in front of their face. As I listened to my medical team
describe our patient's vital signs, the calories she ingested, the level of
sodium in her blood, and other important metrics, I also listened to the
phone. I heard the unmistakable sounds of a popular cartoon about a
city where dogs carry out all of the community's civic functions including policing, construction work, firefighting, air travel, sanitation,
water safety, and the like. I dislike this cartoon, both for the punish-
ingly catchy theme song and the lack of any discernible takeaways from
the stories of the puppies' exploits. Not all children's television needs
to be laden with life teachings, but this show is for me a particularly
saccharine form of entertainment.*

*But here was my patient, just a few weeks old, her future develop-
ment in serious question, facing a television show with questionable
teachable moments. I stopped rounds, interrupting my team, and
turned toward the mother. "What are you watching?" I asked.*

*She said the name of the cartoon. My fears were confirmed. "I
know she's at risk for having issues when she is older," the mother said,
"so I'm just trying to expose her to things kids like so she can grow up
the best she can." Kids do really like that show, but it wasn't the type of
stimulation her newborn needed. Infants can't engage with screens in a
meaningful way.*

*"Wow," I replied, "I can tell you have really been listening to the
NICU team and thinking about how you can help support your baby's
development. That is incredible. We know that at this age infants can't
really engage with television shows, but they can engage with you.
What you are doing, how you are moving, the way you talk. Listening,
learning, being with her, building a relationship with her—that's what
is most important."*

*The mother nodded. Phone still in her baby's face, she wanted to do
the best she could.*

"Do you mind if I grab a book for you from our library? We have a library share here in the NICU and I think you will enjoy reading this book out loud to your baby. Your baby knows and loves your voice [more on this later]. I bet we have one with the dogs in it." Rounds were paused, and I went to find some dog literature with the characters she wanted her baby to know.

The Person You Hope to Raise

Parents often think the use of technology will enrich their child; this is not untrue. I love media and my children engage with it, and it brings us joy and connection. However, technology also can act as a screen, separating us from what really matters for our baby's development: our thoughtful presence. While things like smartphones, tablets, television, and video games are colorful and creative, infants *need* person-to-person engagement to learn and develop. In fact, the American Academy of Pediatrics recommends avoiding most screens—except maybe FaceTime for family communication—for children younger than 2 years. Because the sensory experience of seeing, smelling, hearing, touching, and even tasting caregivers is the ultimate form of nurturing for young children. Responsive, attuned parents help their baby grow smarter and psychologically stronger. That kind of parenting can start at birth.

Let's imagine you are cradling your infant right now, even though you are reading a book about parenting an infant—you could be doing both. Embracing the world of multitasking, take a minute to stop stressing about the life-altering and somewhat fleeting infancy period. Instead, when parenting the newborn, think of the adult you want them to become. What kind of person do you want them to be, and how can you model for them so they can learn? Although their routine might be eat, sleep, poop, build exponential neuronal networks, repeat, yours might be like this: stop, listen, model/guide, repeat.

I didn't imagine the kind of adult I wanted my first child to be, but I wish I had, to help me cope with living with my first newborn. When my daughter was an infant, I'd tell her how pretty she looked, or how good she was when she was quiet and not crying. Then I realized, a quiet pretty woman wasn't a fitting description of me, or really of any woman in my family. I didn't want her to be those things. I wanted her to be free to be her emotional and expressive self. If someone had been asked to describe her in 3 words, I wanted those words to be rare, bold, and wild. Not cute, docile, and fashionable. My hope, my overall goal, was to raise an energetic, kind, and empathetic person.

Reflecting on and imagining the type of person I wanted to raise changed the way I interacted with my daughter. It helped me to look for the nuances of her personality to embrace and understand how to allow her to be her best self. I gave up trying to control her actions and focused on listening to her. Take her 4-month well-child visit. Stranger anxiety for infants generally occurs around 8 to 9 months of age, when a baby prefers their parents and shows some mistrust of strangers. My pediatrician told me that my tiny 4-month-old had all the trappings of stranger anxiety at a young age. She was bright, giggly, and interactive with my husband and me, but the minute she was in front of a stranger she was stone-faced, silent, and suspicious. I wanted others to see the warm and sensitive little baby I knew, but that simply wasn't what she felt like sharing. So, I had to embrace her introverted nature—a very difficult thing for an extroverted people pleaser to do. I also learned not to make excuses for her actions. I would simply say she wasn't interested in talking or playing. Forming a strong relationship with an infant means giving yourself the time and space to observe, as well as the patience to approach them with curiosity and empathy as they learn about the world around them.

New parents often ask me what they can do to support their baby's learning experiences—in essence to expand their baby's brain to help them grow and thrive. My answer is always the same: All they need is a loving and trusting relationship with you. Stop and find a way to listen to their needs and respond to them in the moment. Living from moment to moment is one of the stresses of parenting a newborn. The truth is that what they find extremely stimulating can be super boring for you. Particularly in the beginning, it can feel like a one-sided relationship. But it can also be one of the most overwhelming joys of your life to watch their responses to you grow. Truly listening, though, which, with a newborn, includes using your eyes as much as your ears, is extremely difficult but will pay off. As my little introvert grew, I started to see the activities she was interested in and talking about. I'd encourage those around her to share in her joy of drawing, painting, and swimming. Activities that she more willingly wanted to do with others because they deeply interested her. I had to focus on those things to share with her as she grew. Did I still wish she was bubbly and open and let people into her world easily? Yes, I did. But I can't force her to be what she is not, and I've found a lot more peace and happiness by embracing her temperament and not making excuses for it or trying to mold it.

It's not easy though to sit back and just support my children as they grow, knowing I have little control over their responses to the world around them. I can nurture them and help them understand the world as I see it, but their thoughts and feelings are uniquely their own. That's why when you tell people to just be there for their baby, the easy response is just to say, "Buzz off." It's hard to just be. To not fill your child's life with activities but to sit back, relax, and let them guide you in their wants and needs. Parents want to be told exactly how to fill the time from 1:15 to 1:45 pm in their baby's schedule. Like somehow a half hour of unstructured time will topple the generous neuronal networks the baby is forming.

A packed schedule is the opposite of what you need to parent a newborn. For instance, there is no evidence that listening to Mozart for 30 minutes a day will help your baby get into the best college. Newborns are programmed to get attention from you and respond to you. That attention can be as simple as having them in a baby carrier while you walk around the house doing chores. A simple exchange of touch, sound, and comfort works. The activity you do with a newborn is not as important as your presence. Instead of worrying about a schedule or what is on your to-do list, or needing to do this one activity for your baby to gain IQ points, think about how you can be there for an often unexciting (ok boring) period of time. Are you talking to yourself? That's a great way to get the baby excited. Walking around the house with the baby and loading the drier? It's amazing for the baby to watch and smell your fresh detergent. Your relationship will be built by spending time together, often doing small, mundane activities. This time together will teach the baby how to conduct themselves and help shape their beliefs and attitudes because they will see how you respond to tasks in your everyday life. They will learn your moods and habits and become more attached to you and them—that's what you want. And it will give you time spent together building your long-standing relationship.

Babies Gonna Do

For many years I was guilty of referring to babies as "sacks of potatoes" or "glorified house plants." Because it's hard to know what a baby is thinking and doing every day. Well, again, there is the routine of sleep, eat, poop, build exponential neuronal networks, repeat. Yet, in addition to the monotony of bodily functions your child will exhibit (and then laugh about hysterically at dinner when they turn

3 years old), a more complex development is going on. Things a group of spuds or a vivacious fern could never do.

What is your newborn actually *doing* every day? Your baby's brain is growing at a phenomenal speed. It is making approximately 1 million neuronal connections every second. In the first year after birth, the brain will form billions of nerve pathways and exhibit exponential growth and potential. This is an incredible year for their brain, and its growth will never be as stupendous. You may think, like I do, that getting the laundry done (I mean completely done, folded, and put away) on a weekday or finally taking a dress to the dry cleaner 3 months after wearing it is an incredible feat. However, your newborn has done more in their sleep than you have done in all of your errands in a day. These early connections lay the groundwork for future ones, so the more robust and strong they are, the stronger your child will grow up to be. The budding early connections they are forming are constantly being reduced for efficiency in a process called *pruning*.

Pruning is also used to describe cutting back the leaves and branches of plants. So maybe describing a baby as a house plant isn't entirely off the mark. Let's say a baby is a houseplant; that makes you a gardener. This is a new full-time position for you. Previously, you were not a gardener (a parent) because you didn't have a garden (kids) and, sure, you used to garden as a hobby (babysit, be a cool aunt or uncle), but this is now a calling, a new profession. You probably had all these expectations about gardening, but your experience depends on what you are trying to grow. And plants don't talk. You are going to have to learn how to care for them and help them thrive.

To be a gardener you will need certain tools; your bare hands are only going to help you get so deep. When you investigate gardening materials, you are taken aback by the options. So many different types of pots (cribs), fertilizers (milks), fancy watering cans (peepee teepees); you could spend a ton of money caring for this garden. But what do you truly need to make it flourish? At the end of the day, houseplants need only a few things: soil, sunlight, water, and an optimal climate in which to grow. What does a baby need? One loving, caring, devoted relationship. People are born immature, and a caregiver is required for their survival; we all get that. But a loving attentive caregiver is also *necessary* for their social, emotional, and intellectual growth. It doesn't have to be just one caregiver, though one will do. Caregivers help babies take root in the world and allow their brains to flower. Love is the most powerful fertilizer. You can amass a great toolkit for the care of your child, but ultimately your attention and focus—not on things but on them—will make them flourish.

What's a Parent to Do?

I've only been able to keep a plant alive for a week or two tops. My husband has a little bit more of a green thumb, but our backyard garden is an unruly mess of greenery. We prefer to describe it as "natural." So how do we sow the great fields of our children's minds?

Remember, your newborn's brain is growing and expanding all the time. You don't have to be stressing about it for it to happen. What helps it grow roots (or nerves) are social relationships. Relationships are the water and sun, the key to brain development and growth. Infants can build relationships from the moment they are born. They, like seeds, are not passive. Don't be fooled by the cross-eyed stare you get in the first 6 to 8 weeks after birth. They are constantly receiving emotional responses from you and processing them. How they do that is based on what they see and feel from you and whomever else is devoted to them. The emotional well-being and social experiences of an infant will affect the kind of adult they become. Their emotional health bleeds over into their ability to develop motor, language, and problem-solving skills—relationships grow them. Their social network is not some social media mecca, it's a calm, loving, physical presence.

I mentioned earlier that a lot of parents ask me what they can do to help support their baby's development. They are open to forming a relationship with their baby but worried about doing it "wrong." It's normal to be sensitive and impressionable as a parent, particularly a birth parent coping with the physical challenges and changes of delivering a baby. What works best for your newborn is having someone who responds to and interacts with them. This dynamic interaction is called *serve and return*. Baby smirks, you smile back. Baby babbles, you mush a bunch of vowels together and oooo and aaahhhh at them. Infants need someone to connect with.

If you feel you have a lot of anxiety radiating through your body about how to entertain your infant, give yourself a big hug. Use your energy to just live in the moment with the baby. Start building a dialogue, talk to the baby about what you want for them and let them listen. Eye contact with your baby teaches them trust. Trusting your physical and emotional presence is enough for the baby and one of the best things you can do for them.

Companies and entrepreneurs target new families in big marketing schemes. They will try to sell you on the idea that you need all these toys, videos, or music series to build your baby's brain and make them more intelligent. Like when I mentioned Mozart, none of this is scientifically proven to work in infants.

What is proven is just being with you. I used to have long conversations with my son about the intricacies of loading and unloading the dishwasher. To this day I still cannot get bowls to stack properly in the metal prongs of the washer drawers. Was it stimulating for me to lament about stacking flatware to my newborn? Not really. I felt insane, and still am frustrated that I can't get the bowls to sit properly in the dishwasher. But given that you don't really feel like yourself after having a baby, I went with it. But was it stimulating for my son? Definitely. I shared with my son some of the struggles I was experiencing and let him listen as I tried to find solutions. If you ask my son, he won't remember the detailed hardships I laid out about the dishes. That's ok, though, because I wasn't really trying to "teach" him anything except the fact that he could count on me to interact with. The close contact and steady speech were shaping his neurons. This happens when you just hang out with your baby and talk to them. Hear what I'm saying? We will go over each of the 5 senses and how you can use them to build a strong relationship with your infant.

Hearing

I've stressed the importance of simply talking to your baby. The sense of hearing is well developed in infants right out of the womb. In fact, every baby undergoes a hearing screen soon after birth (see Chapter 5) because it's believed their ears and brain are ready for this sensory skill. So, talk to your baby a lot. Sure, they won't understand and be able to respond, but they will listen, and they are always learning. When they do begin to talk, hearing you speak is going to help them figure out words and phrases. Have conversations with them when they make an utterance that seems like a response to something you said. For example, if you say, "Good morning baby, it's so nice to see you," and they say "coooo," then you coo back—"Coo to you too!" You can begin to imagine what they are saying and let them know that when they speak, someone responds. Play your favorite music, and let them absorb it. This is the fleeting time in childhood when they won't understand any explicit lyrics they shouldn't repeat in public. Embrace—let the expletives fly. Be mindful that some of the songs might be overstimulating, but you don't have to be trapped playing baby shark endlessly to a newborn. With a toddler, I can't promise you they won't gravitate toward memorizing those lyrics, but with a newborn you've still got control of the dial. And don't forget to laugh. One mom told me that when she was pregnant and afterward her goal was to have one great big belly laugh a day.

Laughter might be just what you need when a big poop blows out over the diaper's edge, there is vomit in your hair, or there is urine on your jeans. Kids laugh way more than adults; we need to join them.

Vision

Many times, parents want me to tell them exactly what their infant can see. We can do MRIs (magnetic resonance images) of babies' brains, we can wave things in front of their faces, but we don't really know how they are experiencing the sense of sight except to say most are. We know they can respond to light and dark, which is why you might find the baby staring at your lamp even on day 1. We also know color vision doesn't develop until around 2 to 4 months, so infants may respond more to contrasting shades of black and white than to a colorful rainbow at first. There is a reason why toys for newborns are big explosions of patterned materials. These often bright, shiny, or checkered black and white objects may catch your infant's eye, and trying to look at and follow these objects can be a great way to interact with them. Also, let's face it, your face is very interesting to a baby. Infants learn to differentiate faces early on, starting around the time they get their social smile at 4 to 6 weeks. The faces of loving caregivers make babies go gaga, so make sure you do a lot of face time with your baby. Actual real-life face time. They will love it and their brains will grow.

Smell

Many parents report that their infant smells wonderful. There is something intoxicating about the scent of a newborn. Some pheromonal cue that makes you want to just sniff them all day. Parents report their newborn smell as being sweet, and I swear my infant's stools smelled like fresh yogurt. Babies are playing a sophisticated scent game to make you love them. There is evidence to suggest that how *you* smell is comforting for the baby. Where I work in the NICU parents often leave scent cloths for infants so they can smell the presence of their loving caregiver, even if they can't physically be there with the baby. Don't drench your baby in essential oils or perfumes; relish the sweetness they already have and let them take your sweaty human scents in.

Taste and Touch

Taste is a little tricky because all a baby really needs is the taste of their milk. That said, infants are big oral explorers. You might not think to stick a sweater into your mouth while shopping to decide if you will buy it, but babies often stick everything in there. As babies grow and are sitting in a chair, they want to reach out to taste anything within their grasp. They are experiencing a lot of unique flavors. Be mindful of them only putting safe objects into their mouths, ones with fun textures they can enjoy while teething, not objects that pose a choking risk. Large teething rings without any small beads, various types of pacifiers, and plush toys without detachable eyes or other small plastic features are good examples of safe objects.

Taste and touch are related, and touch is of the utmost importance for a newborn. The NICU recommends something called kangaroo care for newborns. Kangaroos give birth to their little joeys (all their babies are named joey, must be confusing) when they are too small to fend for themselves. So, they go into their mother's pouch to grow and develop. Channeling these marsupial moms might just help your baby better regulate their bodies. By placing an infant on your chest, you are not only comforting them, but you are also helping their body function better. In newborns who need the NICU, this skin-to-skin contact has been known to help them maintain their heart rate and oxygen levels. It has a direct and measurable effect on their physical well-being. If you are out and about and don't feel comfortable having a bare chest as you walk around, consider "baby wearing." The safe way to baby wear is to make sure you can see the baby's face and nose and they are breathing comfortably with their head supported on your chest. You also must make sure to have appropriate hip placement in your baby carrier to facilitate proper development of the hip joint, particularly if you are wearing your baby everywhere. Let the baby's hips and legs straddle your body with the knees apart, and support their thighs. The hips themselves should be bent. Also, don't think you have to hold your baby in a cradle position when walking around without a baby carrier. Try throwing them over your shoulder or supporting them with a hand on their belly. Infants like to try different holding positions; it helps them see the world differently and you might find they enjoy some more than others.

USING THE 5 SENSES FOR INFANT (2–6 MONTH) DEVELOPMENT

SENSE	WAY TO INTERACT WITH BABY
Sight	Bright, shiny, interesting objects for baby to look at
	Infants can't perceive color until ~2–4 months old; use black-and-white contrasted objects for stimulation.
	Show them your face, they will learn it; vary facial expressions.
Hearing	Talk often; let them learn your voice.
	Respond when they talk to you or babble back.
	Let yourself have conversations with your baby, imagine their responses.
	Laugh.
	Play music.
Smell	Your scent can be calming for an infant.
	If separated, consider a scent cloth with your scent to wrap them in as a swaddle.
Taste	Infants like to explore with their mouths; let them.
	Safe textures, small tastes.
Touch	Hold your baby, do skin to skin, this can regulate their temperature and vital signs like heart rate.
	Place your infant in different positions so they can see the world from fun angles.
	Baby wear, keep them close when you walk.

The End of the Innocence

I've listened to a lot of Don Henley to bring you this section of the book. I'm not super old, just kind of old; in my defense Henley is undeniably a catchy '80s rock artist. And you know every love song…ok, really, every song is about my kids now. So "The End of the Innocence" is no different. If you view your infant as a small, frail creature incapable of wrong, innocent, and without a care in the world, don't. Infants are not born fragile or "innocent" because they haven't even learned what it means to be guilty of something. These terms are complex ones that adults understand; infants are just living their lives. They are born naked and exposed to everything with higher-than-you'd-expect levels of processing. They bear witness to their surroundings, and research shows they are a direct product of them, starting at birth. So right when they are born, the end of the innocence has come.

If you haven't heard of adverse childhood experiences (ACEs), the Centers for Disease Control and Prevention offers great resources to describe them. These are potentially traumatic events that occur in childhood, from the newborn period all the way to the teenage years. Examples include substance use or mental health problems in the household, and instability due to things like divorce or incarceration of a parent. The bottom line is that traumatic experiences at any age can impact health, development, and well-being.

An infant's experiences and the relationships cultivated by the adults around them will help shape their entire life. Instead of only focusing on ACEs, many pediatricians have begun promoting PCEs (positive childhood experiences). Relationships are vital to growth and development. Strong, stable, nurturing relationships can determine how a child does in school, their professional opportunities, earning potential, and future partnerships—yeah, all that stuff. Relationships are what make an infant thrive. Even if a family has many

ACEs—and basically all families have some—when parents and caregivers receive support to foster close connections to their babies and incorporate PCEs, this can protect their infants from the trauma of ACEs. Turns out that PCEs may count just as much as adverse experiences in shaping us. No matter the circumstances you find yourself in when you become a parent, focusing on resilience and connectedness and educating yourself about infant development and parenting will help increase the PCEs in your family. The emotional energy you expend when your child is an infant will shape their brain. It's all about love and connection—with yourself and with them. Relationship building early on, responsiveness, and love can be everything.

Physical health and emotional health are tied together, so fortifying early relational health with your newborn is what should truly be on your baby bonding plan. It will help you set the foundation for interacting with the person you have begun to raise.

Chapter 10

Milestone Markers: Visiting Your Pediatrician

*L*et's call the baby in this story Flora. I remember her well. She was a very small baby who was born at 30 weeks, so she was in the neonatal intensive care unit (NICU) because of her prematurity. What made her a unique 30-week infant was her very very small size. Most babies born at 30 weeks weigh around 2½ to 3 pounds, but Flora only weighed around 1½ pounds at birth. This made her look more like a 25-week newborn than a 30-week newborn.

In the NICU, we don't expect infants born before their due dates to do much. They were supposed to be fetuses, and a fetus is constrained in their movements, doesn't have all their reflexes, and needs a calm, dark environment to grow. The NICU is not the relaxing biological environment of the womb; it's a loud, bright, alarm-filled space. So how does the stark change in surroundings affect a preterm baby's growth and development? This is something Flora's mother desperately wanted to know.

Flora's mother is also what made Flora—apart from her petite size—so memorable. She wanted to make sure Flora got every advantage possible to help with her brain growth. Her anxious energy about Flora's progress was something you could feel when you walked up to Flora's bedside. She visited every day—a luxury not all NICU families in the United States have—and her goal was to provide Flora with the stimulation she needed...and then some. However, as neonatologists, we think babies who are as small and premature as Flora need some time to grow before they can tolerate a lot of sound and movement.

We compare an infant's chronological age to their adjusted or corrected age to discuss their developmental needs.

Chronological age = how old you are in days or weeks

Adjusted or corrected age = how you should be acting developmentally

Let's take Flora as an example. She was born at 30 weeks' gesta-tion. When she was 2 months old (8 weeks, her chronological age), we expected her to act like a term infant. Even though she was in fact 2 months old. That is because her adjusted or corrected age was 38 weeks. What developmental stimulus does a 38-week newborn need? They need a caregiver who shows them warmth and affection. We don't expect a lot of tummy time, no cooing sounds, no sustained direct eye contact, and because they don't notice and recognize faces well, no social smile just yet either. In a typical term baby, sure, at 2 months old they begin to exhibit these behaviors, but a preterm baby—no.

When Flora turned 2 months old, her mother took her inability to do what a typical 2-month-old baby does as her falling behind. It crushed her. She pushed for Flora to be out of bed, to be tracking toy objects, to be on her tummy. Flora would protest this, instead favoring the eat, sleep, poop, build exponential neuronal networks, repeat rou-tine of newborns. Flora was still learning to eat because preterm babies take a little bit more time to develop their ability to suck-swallow-breathe than their full-term counterparts. The way Flora would insist she needed rest was by experiencing changes in her vital signs. Her heart rate or oxygen saturation dropped, prompting nurses to remind Flora's mother about the importance of treating her like a newborn and not a 2-month-old.

Can you blame Flora's mother for wanting to push her? Absolutely not. There is a pressure on modern parents to make sure they are doing everything they can to stimulate development. And parents believe they must stimulate their baby or risk them falling behind. Their baby has

to do things first, excel, be a baby trailblazer, and become an amazing achiever all around! But there is more to success than achievement. Babies (and older kids for that matter) follow their own developmental calendar. You can't force a baby to be ready to roll when their body is not. You can make sure they have developmental supports if they aren't rolling by 6 months old, but even at 6 months there is no forcing an infant to bend to your developmental timeline. Parents have to work toward putting wellness above achievement for their little ones as they grow. Parenting isn't about accelerating infant milestones; it's about supporting the baby you have.

Let's Visit the Pediatrician

In a baby's first year, they will have at least 9 appointments with their pediatrician. That's right, *at least 9.* These visits are essential for checking in on a baby's development and helping you to understand typical infant behavior as your baby grows. Your pediatrician is not going to relationship build or parent for you—but they are going to have tips about creating stable, nurturing relationships. They do have the experience of supporting many families and can share all they have learned from helping others.

Week 1

After you leave the hospital, you will visit your pediatrician within 1 to 3 days. The reason for this is to check on the baby's weight and make sure they are getting adequate hydration and calories from their feeds. Babies need this "check-in" for their health and your sanity as you embark on feeding a baby. Some pediatricians will ask you to come back at 7 days (so in a few days) because they want to see if the baby gained weight in the first week. The pediatrician also might ask you to come back on day 14 if they are tracking weights closely.

In terms of development, your newborn should not roll—that's a 6-month-old baby thing. Newborns move their arms and legs and suckle but that's about it. We've talked about fun newborn reflexes (see Chapter 4)—being able to step when held upright, wiggling their bottom, throwing their arms out in a startle—but a newborn's biggest achievements are generally spurts of sleep and telling you when they need to eat.

Month 1

The 1-month visit is again a weight check. Is the baby growing? It's also an important parent check. How does the birth parent feel? Anxious, overwhelmed, tired, proud, elated? So many birth parents only have a 6-week postpartum check for themselves, but the 1-month pediatric visit can also be for you. It's important to know the baby is thriving, but they won't do that well if the family unit isn't thriving too. So, use this as a check-in for everyone. Ask all the questions you have. Your pediatrician is there to answer all of them and address your fears.

Month 2

The 2-month visit is vital. Vital signs are checked, and yes, there is a weight check—always have to be charting where the weight is going. This is the visit, though, where the routine vaccination schedule begins. At this time in a baby's life, the immunity they get from their mother—especially the antibodies or proteins passed on from the placenta—starts to wane. Also, the baby's immune system begins to get strong enough to fight infection. This visit is the start of your preventive care—care you provide for your child that will help them become stronger and healthier. That's exciting, and a little scary. Because they might develop a fever after getting shots, but it's not a freak-out go-to-the-emergency-room fever like they may have had as a newborn. It's a new frontier for their immunity and growth.

At about 2 months, or 8 weeks of age, things also start to get fun developmentally. New skills start to appear. It's when you can start receiving some real feedback on your baby bonding. In the past, pediatricians would talk about reaching milestones on a baby's own timeline—and this is something we still preach. However, we used to refer to different months of a baby's life—say 2, 4, and 6 months— and say that on average half of babies will have this skill. If your baby wasn't in the half that had the skill, we'd say it's cool—wait and see how they develop in the next 2 months.

What we realized is that this approach probably wasn't the most helpful and could be more stressful for families. What if your baby wasn't in the upper half who had the skill? Was there something wrong with your baby? How long did the wait-and-see approach last? Parents wanted answers, and the Centers for Disease Control and Prevention (CDC) and the American Academy of Pediatrics listened and revised developmental milestones for children starting in 2019. The new checklists specify that three-quarters, or 75%, of babies should be displaying these developmental skills. If your baby isn't, it is time to investigate and consider additional screenings or interventions to help them reach their developmental potential. A good pediatrician won't just give you a checklist; they will also ask you open-ended questions about how things are going. The milestones are meant to help you get comfortable sharing your perspectives and making sure you can ask questions or discuss concerns. It opens the door for you to express how you see your baby bonding with you and learning about their environment. And they will offer resources and help if you feel something is amiss. Also, it's nice to get reassurance when your baby is on track, acknowledgment that your baby is doing well even if your stress levels are still high.

The updated milestones checklists on the CDC website are super helpful in knowing what your baby should be achieving. You cannot compare any 2 babies, though; even twins do things differently, and different isn't bad or wrong…it's just different. There is no use comparing your baby with someone else's because how you bond and how your baby grows depend on more than just you and your interactions. I remember my obstetrician teaching me about this. When I was pregnant with my first and second babies, I felt them kicking around a lot, but my third was not as active. In part, I probably didn't feel her as much because my placenta was anterior or right up against the front of my belly and masked some of her movement. I felt her enough not to worry but told my obstetrician she was not as active. She laughed and said I shouldn't compare my kids, and remarked there was still so much I had to figure out once I met her. Because developmental differences and the way and rate in which your child grows by and large don't reflect your parenting. It's a complex mash-up of parenting, environment, resources, and genetics, so one of the only things you can control is making sure you are giving them the resources they need to be on track to achieve and grow. The most important resource is you, and every child is going to need different things, so being open to learning and growing with yours is the key to parenting them well, especially during the newborn period.

2 MONTHS OLD: ANSWER YES/NO TO DOES YOUR INFANT . . .

Calm down when you speak to them or pick them up?

Look at your face?

Seem happy to see you and when you walk up to them?

Smile when you talk to or smile at them?

Make sounds other than crying?

React to loud sounds?

Watch you as your move?

Look at a toy for a few seconds?

Hold their head up when on their tummy?

Move their arms and legs?

Open their hands briefly from a fist?

If you answered "no" to anything, discuss it with your pediatrician.

Adapted from Centers for Disease Control and Prevention. Milestones. Reviewed May 8, 2024. Accessed January 24, 2025. https://www.cdc.gov/ncbddd/actearly/milestones/index.html.

At Least 9 Visits

We are still counting. We have the after-hospital visit, the 1-week visit, the possible 2-week visit, the 1-month visit, and the 2-month visit. That's 4 to 5 visits for the baby and they are just 2 months old. In the first year, remember, they will have around 9 visits. When are the others? Once you hit 2 months, hopefully you will start to space visits every 2 months. That means the next 2 are at 4 and 6 months. For one of my kids, I had to do a 5-month and 7½-month visit for weight checks secondary to breastfeeding issues (tongue-tie, see Chapter 6), so sometimes that spacing doesn't happen. My insurance company and I are likely still talking about covering those visits upon publication of this book, but back to our regularly scheduled visits. To round out the year, you will have a 9-month and a 12-month visit. And then it's time to party because you've gotten a year of care under your belt, an awesome relationship with your pediatrician, and more years to enjoy in the office watching your baby grow and bonding with them.

4 MONTHS OLD: ANSWER YES/NO
TO DOES YOUR BABY . . .

Smile to get your attention?

Laugh when you try to make them?

Look at you, move, or make sounds to get your attention?

Make oooo, ahhh, and cooing noises?

Make sounds back when you chat with them?

Turn their head to the sound of your voice?

When hungry and they see milk, open their mouth to get it?

Look at their hands. I mean really look at them with interest?

Hold their head steady without support when being held?

Hold a toy when it's put in their hand?

Use their arms to swipe or swing at toys?

Bring their hands up to their mouth?

Push up on their elbows or forearms when on their tummy?

If you answered "no" to anything above, your pediatrician will want to discuss this with you and find out more information.

6 MONTHS OLD: ANSWER YES/NO
TO DOES YOUR BABY . . .

Know familiar people?

Look at themselves in the mirror?

Laugh?

Take turns making sounds with you?

Do raspberries? Not eat them, but blow them at you? (Who doesn't love a wet kiss?)

Make squealing noises?

Put things in their mouth to explore?

Reach to grab a toy when they want one?

Close their lips or turn away when they don't want food or milk?

Roll from their tummy to their back?

Push up with straight arms when they are on their tummy?

Lean on their hands and try to sit?

If you answered "no" to anything, your pediatrician will want to discuss this with you and find out more information.

Adapted from Centers for Disease Control and Prevention. Milestones. Reviewed May 8, 2024. Accessed January 24, 2025. https://www.cdc.gov/ncbddd/actearly/milestones/index.html.

For more information on 9-month and 12-month developmental milestones and others from the CDC please use this QR code.

Chapter 11

Baby Bonding

T hrough real stories from the neonatal intensive care unit and my own personal experiences, I hope I've shown you that infants are capable of complex relationships from the moment they are born and how you can ensure their health and safety to build those relationships. They have real emotions and are not houseplants or sacks of potatoes. Babies are immature humans who need your love to grow and thrive. And you will be surprised how quickly this will happen. The first few years of their lives are the most remarkable, as they set up the framework and foundation of their brains. At a time of rapid change, your relationship is required as a constant grounding presence.

We don't hear a lot about an infant's mental health, as you can't screen a baby with a questionnaire or ask them if they are feeling happy or sad. But as a neonatologist and pediatrician I feel confident an infant will thrive when they have safe, stable, nurturing relationships to help them grow, and we have an acronym for this: SSNR. Their physical well-being depends on conscientious open-hearted caregivers. A sense of who they are and the confidence needed to approach the world grow from SSNR. There is no one-size-fits-all formula for how to form this bond and support your infant, but there are strategies you can follow to plant the seeds for future stability and independence. Creating your baby bonding plan and following it will help guide you to become the safe, stable, nurturing parent your infant needs; let's give you steps to get there and stay there as you parent.

Being Safe...

What does it mean to a baby to feel safe? Safety itself is when someone feels free from fear and that their environment won't hurt them. People can feel hurt both physically and emotionally, so as the parent of a newborn you are responsible for both the physical and psychological safety of your baby.

Physical Safety

The physical safety of your baby sounds straightforward. You want to make sure your baby is in an environment in which they can't hurt themselves. The plus side to having a newborn is they really can't move much. When you put them down on a flat surface, they generally stay put.

Physical safety becomes harder to attain when they really get crawling, cruising, and walking—maybe my next book will be about babyproofing your house. That's why pediatricians emphasize safe sleep so much—because being in a safe environment for sleep when they are under less supervision is so important. Don't leave your baby in a crib with an inclined surface. Don't leave any plush toys, pillows, blankets, or bumper pads in their crib. You do not want any soft and suffocating objects in the crib when you aren't around to watch. And ensure that their toys are age appropriate and not something that could smush them or be swallowed.

As a pediatrician, but also a mom, I think of physical safety as also making sure I am tracking their health and development with my own pediatrician. It may sound funny, but a pediatrician needs another pediatrician to watch over their baby because being a parent and being a doctor are entirely different roles. A good doctor has a logical evidenced-based framework with which to treat their patients, while a parent has intuition and a ton of emotion and love that is present when they have to deal with any illness or accident their child might have. So having a pediatrician as a sounding board is a must, even for pediatricians. It's very hard to be calm, collected, and caring when its your baby that cuts their chin and it bleeds a lot, or they have a bad cold and you are sucking mucus out of their nose, tracking their fevers, and watching them breathe with worry. Watching out for their health is many times wrapped into their physical safety. This is also an important section to remember that doing things like vaccinating your child is protecting them physically. That is the part of engaging in routine care that is so essential.

Psychological Safety

Psychological safety for adults can be defined as the ability to interact with others and say what you really feel and mean without fear that something bad will happen to you. The same definition applies to a baby. An infant wants to express themselves and be heard; they want to have someone respond to them. When your infant cries and you don't respond regularly to their needs, it can make them feel less safe. Does that mean you have to jump up every time the baby cries? No. But it means when they call you it's good to have a way to respond to them (refer to "The Cry Baby Checklist" in Chapter 8). The truth is that blips of inattention and underwhelming affection inform creativity, self-care, resilience, and problem-solving skills. You don't need to be "on call" every second. It's about cultivating an overall mood of sensitivity and empathy. You will not and cannot get it right all the time, but you can center yourself and practice sensitive parenting.

Sensitive Parenting

What is sensitive parenting? Let's say your baby is in a crying fit. You've gone through the checklist: feeding, changing, giving them a pacifier, swaddling, swaying, shushing—none of it is working. It is a stressful situation, and you feel like you are about to lose it. Might be time to just check out and hand the baby to another loving caregiver. Or you take a deep breath. You tell the baby it's ok, you tried your best and wish you could make them stop crying and figure out why they are so sad or anger or annoyed. Whatever they are feeling is fine; you acknowledge their feelings and your own feelings, and you stay with them rocking them into the night. Tell them you'll be there for them. Find the space to love with little understanding and little sleep. A sensitive parent responds to their infant's cues in a thoughtful way, expressing empathy toward their experiences. Sensitive parents can literally grow their babies' brains. When researchers conducted studies looking at the brains of children with attuned caregivers, they found increased brain size overall and thicker areas of the brain that allow for problem-solving, thought, and emotional regulation. This bigger brain leads to more secure attachments for these children in the future, so better relationships all around. It also leads to being smarter and more competent and having fewer psychological problems in the future.

...Stable...

Since I mentioned secure attachments, let's talk more about how to introduce stability into your baby's life. To have stability is to have a degree of predictability and consistency in an emotional and physical environment. Children, and this includes babies, really enjoy predictability. They like schedules and patterns and planning. As someone who spent 32 years flying by the seat of my pants in medicine, I found that having a baby was a rock of stability in my life I just wasn't used to. Last-minute decision to go out to an exercise class or dinner with a friend? That's no longer a luxury in my life with a baby. Stability in an infant's life means a certain grounding in

a parent. Making the adjustment to parenting a newborn is challenging because what fills their day isn't necessarily what you would want
to fill yours (re: it can feel really boring). So you have to adjust and
find the joy in sharing the day with someone whose preferences may
differ from yours.

...and Nurturing

To nurture is to give your baby consistent developmental, emotional,
and physical stimulation in a sensitive manner. Are you going to
respond in an incredible brain-boosting way during every moment
of your infant's growth and development? No. You do your best to
provide safety and stability and then you work on nurturing them in
the best ways you know how. Parenting is learning and growing with
your baby.

One great way to nurture is by listening when your baby has
something to say. As your child grows you can begin to encourage
their talents and interests and help them set goals and succeed. But
with an infant, it's more about learning about them and figuring
out their temperament and needs. They are trying to communicate
with you in eye blinks, grunts, cries, and blow-out poops. Some
parents think it isn't until your baby gives you that social smile at 6
to 8 weeks that they are inviting you in to interact with them. But
they want you to interact with them and nurture them from the very
beginning. They need you. Even before they develop any social cues
or language, they are developing the foundation for them. Their little
eyes are seeing more and more, and your face is their map of the
world. They will read your nonverbal cues and the emotional context
in which you approach them. So even if you aren't trying to communicate with them, you are. They are reading into everything you say
and do. When they make an overture, make one back. This will get
more sophisticated with time, so maybe it starts out that they fart

and cry and then you change their diaper. That's a win in the communications category and a great way to nurture them.

Remember that when your baby cries, you should respond to them. Part of nurturing an infant is providing comfort to help them feel better. It doesn't spoil them; it teaches them that someone will respond to their needs and they can trust you.

The best way to nurture your baby though is to have fun with them. Play is a fundamental part of human growth and development—it's not frivolous or something to do only when you have extra time. What counts as play? Play can be loosely defined as taking part in an activity for enjoyment or recreation and not for a practical purpose. Think of play as an activity that doesn't require a lot of thought, that engages you, and that allows for joyful discovery. It should be fun and spontaneous. Becoming attuned to your infant and their needs is a form of play. You don't know what to expect, you (and they) don't know what they will do in the next minute, and you respond and try to find happiness and joy in those simple interactions. This back and forth with your baby will help motivate them to learn and grow.

Put laughter as a daily part of your baby bonding plan. Or find a new sound your baby can make, or a new position in which they can place their fingers, hands, or arms. Show interest in them and set aside unstructured portions of the day to just be with them without a cell phone, an errand, or another task. The precious time you get with your infant is laying the foundation for your lifelong relationship together.

Relationship Building and Baby Bonding

It is through relationships that we learn who we are, and that is how we become individuals. An infant's relationship with a loving, trusted caregiver is their first and often most powerful relationship. Safe, stable, nurturing relationships build brains and people. Learning about your baby and adapting your responses to them is a form of social engagement that will help them grow physically and emotionally. It will affect how their heart beats, how their brain forms, and what hormones they release when they are happy, mad, or sad.

While language and its development are important, your connection with your infant starts with nonverbal communication. You learn to harmonize and find synchrony in your responses to life without even speaking. Maybe it's just how you look at them, how you modulate your voice, or the ways in which they watch you engage with your environment that will be key to how their brain forms and how they regulate themselves.

You don't need me to build an actual baby bonding plan with you—you need to do it with your baby. I have provided you with the foundational framework that will guide you to begin to create the groundwork for a plan that is most important to you as a new parent. Whether your baby is still in the womb, just born, or a few months old—begin to think about who you want them to become, what it means for you to parent, and how you can empathize with someone who communicates in cries. These are monumental tasks that you won't be able to complete in one sitting. Not having all the answers or a checklist to complete is ok; in fact, in relationship building and bonding it's probably the best thing for you. Your baby is going to be a new, exciting journey of discovery and you don't need to get a plane ticket to experience it. Everything you need to be an amazing parent is already in your heart. So get out of your head and get in touch with your baby.

Index